OXFORD MED

Dementia care

OXFORD MEDICAL PUBLICATIONS

Dementia care

Contents

Contents

Preface

Cognitive disorders are one of the great challenges of our age.

They are common. Each of us expecting to reach our 80th year has a one in five chance of becoming demented. Manifestations emerge from a spectrum of normal variation in the population, from ability to remember, to behaviour and personality traits. They raise difficult questions about independence and autonomy, coping and caring. They run counter to the expectations of our culture, for strength and wisdom amongst adults. This leads to unfortunate references to 'second childhood' and a whole 'malignant social psychology' of how we treat people with dementia, which exacerbates the very problems that lead to the term being used in the first place. Families and health and social care organizations struggle to cope with people who push at the boundaries of expectation and care provision, leading to frustration, stress, and despair.

Many cognitive disorders are incurable, progressive, and disabling. There is no denying that in some cases dementia can be a miserable condition. But, as with many difficult problems, there is a good way and a bad way of managing it. The good way spots reversible elements and treats them (and in some cases provides an alternative, and sometimes curable, diagnosis). The good way minimizes problems, maximizes function, increases choices, gives information, and supports carers. The bad way leads to unnecessary distress and disability, dissatisfied carers and professionals, excessive institutionalization, prolonged hospital stays, and cost.

These are problems that no adult health or social care professional can avoid. They are everyone's problem. The good news is that there is an expertise that makes a difference.

Do not expect every piece of advice in this book to be backed up by evidence from a randomized, controlled trial. Elderly people, psychiatric disorders, and dementia and delirium have been particularly poorly served by trials. Where there is evidence we need to be aware of it and take account of it. A lot of what we say derives from the accumulated wisdom of people who have reflected intelligently on successful (and sometimes unsuccessful) services. But we believe that what is in this book is worth knowing. Above all it is intended as useful practical advice.

There is now great concern about the harm that sedative drugs can do to people with dementia. Many people would like to see them banned completely, but there is little in the way of effective alternatives in urgent situations. We have tried to indicate how to avoid such crises arising and how to deal with long-term problems, but we have also included guidance on the safe and appropriate use of medication.

The wisdom is multidisciplinary. Whilst doctors have a particular role in making diagnoses and conveying explanations to others, many valuable strands of thought and experience come from nursing and psychology, as well as many other disciplines. We thank Lyndsey Beck, Louise Bevan, Phil Blatherwick, Hilary Cobb, Peter Connelly, Adam Gordon, Kate Gordon, Dawn Newman, Stephanie Page, Mary Read, Lisa Stanton, Pat Sumner, Mary Watson, and Lauren Wintrip, who have advised us on some of these, but of course we take responsibility for the final product and any errors that remain. Special thanks are due to Dorothee Auer and Jim Lowe for images of dementia.

You can read this book from cover to cover, but will probably find it more useful to use as a reference guide on specific issues and topics as they arise.

Abbreviations

6-CIT	6 item Cognitive Impairment Test
A&E	Accident and Emergency
Aβ	Amyloid beta protein
ABC	Antecedents, Behaviours, Consequences
ACE	Angiotensin converting enzyme
AChEI	acetylcholinesterase inhibitor
AD	Alzheimer's disease
AF	Atrial fibrillation
ADAS-Cog	Cognitive subscale of the Alzheimer' Disease Assessment Schedule
ADH	Anti-diuretic hormone
ADL	Activities of daily living
AIDS	Acquired immune deficiency syndrome
AMHP	Approved Mental Health Professional
AMT	Abbreviated mental test
ANH	Artificial nutrition and hydration
APP	Amyloid precursor protein
AWI	Adults with Incapacity (Scotland) Act
bd	twice daily
BMA	British Medical Association
BME	Black and minority ethnic
BNF	British National Formulary
BPSD	Behavioural and psychological symptoms in dementia
BPVS	British Picture Vocabulary Test
C	Celsius
CBD	Cortico-basal degeneration
CBT	Cognitive behavioural therapy
CEA	Carcino-embryonic antigen
CI	Confidence interval
CJD	Creutzfeldt-Jakob disease
CK	Creatine kinase
CMHT	Community mental health team
COMT	Catechol-o-methyl transferase
COPD	Chronic obstructive pulmonary disease
CPN	Community psychiatric nurse
CPR	Cardio-pulmonary resuscitation
CRP	C-reactive protein

CSF	Cerebro-spinal fluid
CSCI	Commission for Social Care Inspection
CST	Cognitive stimulation therapy
CT	Computed tomography
CXR	Chest X-ray
d	day
DCM	Dementia Care Mapping
DLB	Dementia with Lewy Bodies
DMR	Dementia Questionnaire for Mentally Retarded Persons
DoLS	Deprivation of Liberty Safeguards
DSDS	Dementia Scale for Down's Syndrome
DSM-IV	Diagnostic & Statistical Manual 4th edition
DT	Delirium tremens
DVLA	Driver and Vehicle Licensing Authority
DVT	Deep venous thrombosis
ECG	Electrocardiogram
ECHR	European Convention of Human Rights
EEG	Electroencephalogram
EPA	Enduring Power of Attorney
ESR	Erythrocyte sedimentation rate
EU	European Union
FTD	Fronto-temporal dementia
GHQ	General Health Questionnaire
GI	Gastro-intestinal
GP	General practitioner
GPCOG	GP assessment of cognition
h	hour
HAART	Highly active anti-retroviral therapy
HAD	HIV associated dementia
HIV	Human immunodeficiency virus
HRT	Hormone Replacement Therapy
HSV	Herpes simplex virus
ICD	International classification of diseases
im	intramuscular
IMCA	Independent Mental Capacity Advocate
IU	International unit
iv	intra-venous
ITU	Intensive therapy unit
LACL	Large Allen Cognitive Levels
LD	Learning disability

LDL	Low density lipoprotein
LP	Lumbar puncture
LPA	Lasting power of attorney
MAO-B	Monoamine oxidase B
MCA	Mental Capacity Act
mcg	microgram
MCI	Mild cognitive impairment
MCMD	Minor cognitive motor disorder
MEAMS	Middlesex Elderly Assessment of Mental State
mg	milligram
MHA	Mental Health Act
ml	millilitre
MHCTSA	Mental Health (Care and Treatment) (Scotland) Act
MID	Multi-infarct dementia
MMSE	Mini-Mental State Examination
MND	Motor neuron disease
MR	Modified release
MRI	Magnetic resonance imaging
MS	Multiple sclerosis
NAID	Neuropsychological Assessment of Dementia in Individuals with Intellectual Disabilities
NHS	National Health Service
NICE	National Institute for Clinical Excellence
NMDA	n-methyl-d-aspartate
NMS	Neuroleptic malignant syndrome
nmol	nanomole
NPI	Neuropsychiatric inventory
NSAID	Non-steroidal anti-inflammatory drug
nocte	at night
od	once daily
OPG	Office of the Public Guardian
OR	Odds ratio
OT	Occupational therapy (therapist)
PCC	Person centred care
PDD	Parkinson's disease dementia
PE	Pulmonary embolism
PEG	Percutaneous endoscopic gastrostomy
po	*per os* (by mouth)
prn	(as required)
PSA	Prostate specific antigen
PSP	Progressive supranuclear palsy

PTH	Parathyroid hormone
qds	Four times daily
RCN	Royal College of Nursing
RCT	Randomised controlled trial
RO	Reality orientation
RR	Relative risk
s.	section
SALT	Speech and Language Therapist
sc	subcutaneous
SDSA	Stroke driver's screening assessment
SI	Système internationale
SIADH	Syndrome of inappropriate ADH secretion
SLE	Systemic lupus erythematosus
SPECT	Single photon emission computed tomography
SSRI	Selective serotonin re-uptake inhibitor
SVT	supraventricular tachycardia
TB	Tuberculosis
TCA	Tricyclic antidepressant
tds	three times daily
TENS	Transcutaneous electrical nerve stimulation
TGA	Transient global amnesia
TIA	Transient ischaemic attack
TICS	Telephone interview for cognitive status
TSH	Thyroid stimulating hormone
TURP	Transurethral resection of the prostate
U & E	Urea, creatinine and electrolytes
US	Ultrasound
UTI	Urinary tract infection
VA	Visual acuity
VaD	Vascular dementia
VT	ventricular tachycardia
WHO	World Health Organisation

Chapter 1

What is dementia?

Features of dementia

Box 1.1 A definition of dementia

Dementia is an acquired global impairment of intellect, memory and personality but without impairment of consciousness. As such it is almost always of long duration, usually progressive and often irreversible, but these features are not included as part of the definition (Lishman).

The definition in Box 1.1 is convenient and concise but has its limitations. No one is likely to mistake the signs of advanced dementia, but there is always difficulty deciding at what point someone who has been showing gradually worsening memory can be diagnosed as having definite dementia.

No reliable scanning technique or laboratory test can confirm the diagnosis, which is down to the individual judgement of a clinician. Tests can help (📖 Chapter 2), and there are operational criteria for mild, moderate and severe dementia (📖 Box 1.2), but the earlier the diagnosis of dementia is made, the more uncertain it will be. WHO criteria require symptoms to be present for at least 6 months, and specify that the impairment is 'sufficient to interfere with everyday activities', but people vary greatly in the level of activity they undertake and their ability to cope with declining memory.

There may be remarkable preservation of personality, and initially little in the way of intellectual impairment apart from memory loss, particularly in very elderly people. Where personality changes do occur, they usually take the form of an exaggeration of previous character traits. People with dementia easily develop delirium (📖 Chapter 3), and in such circumstances a degree of impairment of consciousness is likely. In dementia with Lewy bodies (DLB), clouding of consciousness and psychotic symptoms such as hallucinations and delusions may be a prominent feature even in the absence of any acute illness to cause delirium.

In the majority of cases onset is insidious, with gradual slow deterioration. If the onset is abrupt or memory loss is not the first symptom, the diagnosis is almost certainly not dementia, although strokes and head injuries can cause a sudden onset of irreversible cognitive impairment. Sometimes the first presentation of dementia is with 'delirium' that does not completely resolve (📖 Chapters 3 and 8).

Box 1.2 General criteria for dementia (after WHO ICD-10 Diagnostic Criteria for Research)

- **Decline in memory**
  - Mild—Sufficient to interfere with everyday activities but not to preclude independent living. Problems mostly with learning new material. Difficulty taking in, retaining and recalling matters of everyday life, such as where things have been put, social arrangements or information from family.
  - Moderate—Memory loss a serious handicap to everyday living. Only very familiar material retained. New information retained only occasionally or briefly. Unable to recall basic information on local geography, recent activities and names of familiar people.
  - Severe—Complete inability to learn new information. Only fragments of previously learned information remain. Can't recognize even close relatives.
- **Decline in other cognitive functions:**
  e.g. judgement and thinking, planning and reasoning, processing of information.
  - Mild—Impaired performance in activities of daily living (ADL), but not to a degree that makes the individual dependent on others. Complicated tasks cannot be undertaken.
  - Moderate—Unable to function in ADL without the assistance of another. Only simple chores can be performed. Activities are restricted and poorly sustained.
  - Severe—There is an absence (or virtual absence) of intelligible ideas.
- **Awareness of the environment**
  Absence of clouding of consciousness to permit memory decline to be assessed. Where there is superimposed delirium, the diagnosis of dementia should be deferred.
- **Decline in emotional control and motivation**
  - emotional lability
  - irritability
  - apathy
  - coarsening of social behaviour.
- **Duration**
  The symptoms must be present for 6 months for a confident diagnosis.

Symptoms of dementia

Forgetfulness

The cardinal symptom of dementia is difficulty in taking in and retaining new information, although this may not be the symptom that brings the patient to the attention of services. Memory for recent events is affected first, and as the disease progresses, gradually earlier events in the patient's life are also forgotten; memory for childhood and early life are usually best preserved. People with dementia are generally aware that they are liable to forget things, but tend to minimize the importance of this. Some people with dementia are adept at making up plausible accounts to cover for their failing memories; you should always corroborate details with a reliable informant. Remember, memory loss must be sufficiently severe to interfere with everyday activities.

On occasion family members or the person with symptoms may become unduly concerned about minor memory impairment; it is generally easy to tell when this is happening, but every case of dementia starts with trivial symptoms and you can never guarantee the future course of an illness. It is always worth offering the opportunity of follow-up to check the progression of symptoms.

There are many short screening tests to detect memory loss (📖 Chapter 13 p. 322–325).

Other presentations

In most cases of dementia memory loss is the initial symptom; the remainder may present with psychotic symptoms (particularly in cases of dementia with Lewy bodies, 📖 p. 10–11), personality change (particularly in fronto-temporal dementia, 📖 Chapter 15), other cognitive impairments, or depression. There are clinically relevant differences in dementia in younger people (by convention those under 65, 📖 Chapter 14).

Other impairments of cognition

As dementia progresses, all areas of cognitive functioning can become impaired. It is important to establish from an informant that there has been a decline from a previous level, the commonest misdiagnosis for dementia being long standing borderline learning disability.

Disorientation

Disorientation in time and place is a common early symptom, but is not specific to dementia. It may be due to impaired attention (e.g. in delirium) or memory.

Visuo-spatial problems

After memory loss the next symptoms to appear are generally impairments of visuo-spatial ability. In the clinical setting, early difficulties in this area may be detected by using the clock drawing test, or the intersecting pentagons item from the MMSE (📖 Chapter 13).

Dyspraxia

Dyspraxia is the impairment of the ability to manipulate objects in the absence of gross motor or sensory loss. The term apraxia is sometimes

used; there is no important difference in their meaning. Common examples would include difficulty using household devices e.g.:
• Not being able to use the remote control on a television set.
• Problems with a new kitchen appliance—such as a microwave oven or washing machine.
As dementia progresses, more established skills may be lost e.g.:
• Shaving.
• Inability to put on clothes—either back to front or in the wrong order.

Language problems—dysphasia

Dysphasia (or aphasia) is impairment of the ability to express thought in words (expressive dysphasia), or inability to comprehend what is said or written by others (receptive dysphasia).

The earliest sign of dysphasia in dementia is word finding difficulty—particularly names of things (nominal dysphasia). Where language problems occur in dementia there are usually problems in expressive, receptive and naming aspects (📖 Chapter 4 p. 85–87).

Speech and language difficulties are often present in vascular dementia (📖 p. 8), but early dysphasia in the absence of other focal neurological signs suggests either a stroke or one of the more unusual causes of dementia (📖 Chapter 15 p. 354).

Executive problems ('dysexecutive syndrome')

'Executive functioning' includes a wide variety of activities such as maintaining attention, setting goals, developing plans, modifying plans in response to circumstances, using judgement, inhibiting inappropriate behaviour, and promoting socially acceptable behaviour. Impairments in this area may contribute to dyspraxia by causing difficulty in doing things in a logical sequence. This might include getting dressed correctly, or making a hot drink. Tests to evaluate these difficulties can be found in Chapter 13 (📖 p. 326).

Executive problems often cause problems in undertaking activities of daily living; assessment by an occupational therapist (📖 Chapter 5 p. 112) may be more helpful than undertaking neuropsychological testing.

Behaviour changes

Memory loss is the cardinal feature of dementia, but problems with behaviour cause the greatest distress to carers. Behaviour changes occur at some time during the course of the disorder in about 65% of people with dementia. They most commonly emerge in the middle stages of the disorder, although they may be present from the outset (📖 Chapter 4).

Personality changes

Strictly personality isn't behaviour. By personality we mean a set of traits, habits, or reactions that typify how a person functions day to day.

Personality change is generally a late feature of dementia. It is unusual for people's characters to change dramatically; where this occurs it is usually a result of distress, such as physical pain or mental anguish, which needs further evaluation (📖 Chapter 6 p. 152–4).

More common is the exaggeration of previous personality characteristics: 'They're the same as they always were only more so.'

Some people spend their lives restraining less acceptable aspects of their personality—such as their aggression or sexuality. As dementia progresses these traits may become more overt.

Exacerbation of dementia

Although dementia is a neurological disorder with clear pathological changes (📖 Chapter 16), its manifestations are made worse by many factors. It may first become apparent when away from home, on shopping trips or on holiday, or at a time of physical illness (📖 Chapter 3). The symptoms and signs of the illness may be amplified by the reactions of others to the person with dementia. Developing signs of dementia does not make an adult into a child. Memory may be impaired but important skills and attributes are retained. Appropriate responses to people with dementia can maintain cognitive abilities as well as personal dignity.

Remember that there is a very real possibility that any one of us may develop dementia when we are older—think about how you would wish to be treated.

Causes of dementia

The common causes of dementia are listed in Table 1.1. Dementia is predominantly a disorder of older people. In people under 65, rarer causes of dementia also need to be considered (📖 Chapters 14 and 15).

Alzheimer's disease

This is the commonest cause of dementia in people over 35 in Western countries. The onset is insidious and the progression of symptoms is steady. Memory loss is the most prominent symptom, but older people with Alzheimer's disease (AD) are often remarkably unperturbed by their forgetfulness. This lack of concern is sometimes attributed to lack of insight; most commonly patients are well aware of their memory loss but are content to put it down to normal ageing processes. The pathological features of AD are essentially an exaggeration of normal ageing changes in the brain (📖 Chapter 16), and the symptoms can be understood in the same way. There is no rigid dividing line between normal ageing and AD, which means that giving a definite diagnosis early in the course of the disorder is fraught with difficulties—although families in particular are very eager for this. There is no specific laboratory test for AD; the diagnosis depends on obtaining a typical history and excluding other possible causes for the symptoms (📖 Chapter 2).

A diagnosis of AD requires both symptoms of cognitive impairment and interference with activities of daily living; forgetfulness that does not cause day to day problems is labelled 'mild cognitive impairment' (📖 page 12).

Vascular dementia

Damage to the brain as a result of strokes or disease of cerebral blood vessels may cause dementia. This the second commonest cause after AD (📖 Table 1.1). The features of vascular dementia (VaD) vary depending on whether the condition results from one or more strokes (caused by occlusion of a large vessel or cerebral haemorrhage)—sometimes known as multi-infarct dementia (MID)—or from disease of smaller cerebral vessels. The clinical features that differentiate VaD from AD are listed in Box 1.3.

In small vessel disease the onset is less abrupt than in MID; general slowing of thinking and movement is often prominent. Sometimes when people with this type of dementia respond to questions they can be extraordinarily slow in responding, even when they know the correct answer.

Affective symptoms are common in people with VaD. The condition of 'pathological emotionalism' is particularly distressing. In this disorder people are easily moved to extremes of emotion, outbursts of weeping, or, less frequently, anger provoked by relatively trivial stimuli. The condition may be triggered by a stroke and often resolves spontaneously. If it is distressing or persists, treatment with antidepressant medication (📖 Chapter 6 p. 164) usually helps.

It is sometimes said that there is better preservation of insight in people with VaD. They are certainly more likely to show distress when they cannot perform as well as they wish. People with AD seem more inclined to shrug off their poor memories and attribute difficulties to an inevitable process of ageing, whereas those with VaD are often acutely sensitive to their shortcomings.

Mixed Alzheimer's and vascular dementia

In clinical practice there is a large overlap between Alzheimer's and vascular dementias. Only 20% of patients clinically diagnosed as having AD have no concomitant cerebrovascular disease, and only 5% of those diagnosed with VaD have none of the pathological hallmarks of AD (📖 Chapter 16). This means that not only may people with evidence of vascular disease on a brain scan benefit from cholinesterase inhibitor medication, but also that it is worthwhile trying to reduce vascular risks in people with AD.

Table 1.1 Causes of dementia

Cause	Percentage
Alzheimer's disease	55%
Vascular dementia (includes mixed Alzheimer's and vascular dementia)	20%
Dementia with Lewy bodies	15%
Fronto-temporal dementia	5%
Other causes (see Chapter 15)	5%

Box 1.3 Features of vascular dementia

- Sudden onset of cognitive impairment associated with neurological signs of stroke.
- Fluctuating course of illness; rapid deterioration followed by periods of gradual improvement ('stepwise deterioration').
- History or signs of vascular disease:
  - hypertension
  - ischaemic heart disease
  - peripheral vascular disease
  - stroke.
- Focal neurological signs and symptoms.
- Pathological emotionalism.

Dementia with Lewy bodies and Parkinson's disease dementia

Dementia with Lewy bodies (DLB) is the third commonest form of dementia and may present in many different ways. It is important to recognize DLB, as treating hallucinations and delusions in these patients with antipsychotic medication may cause severe Parkinsonian reactions. The commonest symptoms are listed in Box 1.4.

In DLB there are dramatic biochemical changes in the brain and impairment of cerebral function (demonstrable on EEG) but very little structural damage. Correcting the biochemical changes with appropriate medication (Chapter 6 p. 140) often results in dramatic improvement.

Similar symptoms may occur late in the course of Parkinson's disease. Where the onset of psychological symptoms is more than one year after the onset of motor symptoms of Parkinsonism, the disorder is labelled Parkinson's disease dementia (PDD).

Symptoms in DLB

Diagnosis of DLB can be quite straightforward if the typical features of confusion, psychosis, and Parkinsonism are all present. However, all sorts of presentations are possible. Dramatic neuropsychiatric changes with gross EEG changes but normal CT or MRI imaging are very suggestive of DLB. If you can't work out what the diagnosis is with an unusual case of confusion—it's usually DLB.

Box 1.4 Clinical features of dementia with Lewy bodies (DLB)

- Cognitive impairment:
  - in the early stages memory loss may not be prominent, but this usually occurs as the disorder progresses
  - fluctuations in the level of impairment are common
  - dyspraxia and dysexecutive problems are frequently early symptoms.
- Abnormalities of attention and arousal:
  - clouding of consciousness
  - falling asleep suddenly, difficulty in waking.
- Psychosis:
  - visual hallucinations
  - paranoid auditory hallucinations—may be typical of schizophrenia
  - olfactory and tactile hallucinations (rare)
  - paranoid delusions
  - other systematized delusions.
- Parkinsonism:
  - typical motor features of idiopathic Parkinson's disease
  - even if spontaneous extrapyramidal signs are absent, there may be dramatic side effects from even atypical antipsychotic medication ('neuroleptic sensitivity').
- Associated features:
  - REM sleep behaviour disorder
  - repeated falls and syncope
  - transient unexplained loss of consciousness
  - severe autonomic dysfunction
  - depression.
- Findings on investigation:
  - relatively normal appearances on CT/MRI scans
  - low ligand uptake in the basal ganglia on SPECT imaging
  - prominent slow wave activity on EEG with temporal sharp waves.
- A diagnosis of DLB is less likely in the presence of:
  - stroke disease, either as focal neurological signs or on scanning
  - any other physical illness or brain disorder sufficient to account in part or in total for the clinical picture
  - Parkinsonism only appearing for the first time at a stage of severe dementia.

Mild cognitive impairment

Dementia is a condition of cognitive impairment that is sufficiently severe as to interfere with functional abilities and possibly also with emotions, motivation and social behaviour. There is a state between this and normal ageing, in which there is a decline from a previous level of functioning but not to an extent sufficient to fulfil criteria for dementia. This state is now referred to as mild cognitive impairment (MCI).

This is defined as:

"A syndrome characterized by cognitive decline greater than that expected for an individual's age and education level, which does not interfere notably with activities of daily living. It is not a diagnosis of dementia of any type, although it may lead to dementia in some cases."

Several types of MCI have been described, according to the predominant symptoms present. Amnestic MCI denotes the condition where impairment of memory is the main symptom. About 15% of cases of MCI are likely to progress to dementia each year. It had been hoped that treating MCI might be helpful in preventing the development of dementia, but treatment with cholinesterase inhibitors in amnestic MCI has been shown not to be beneficial.

cohol and dementia

ght-to-moderate consumption of alcohol is beneficial in maintaining ognitive functioning (📖 Chapter 17 Box 17.4), but excessive drinking increases the risk of dementia. Part of this increased risk is due to associated vitamin deficiency causing Wernicke's encephalopathy (📖 Chapter 3 p. 67) and the associated long-term state, Korsakoff's syndrome.

However, prolonged heavy drinking may itself cause cognitive impairment by a direct neurotoxic effect, accompanied by cerebral atrophy, which is at least partially reversible on cessation of alcohol intake. Some estimates suggest that alcohol excess plays a part in up to 10% of people with dementia. Indeed, heavy drinkers with no signs of dementia are often found to have cerebral atrophy on imaging and impairments on neuropsychological testing. People who drink too much are also liable to head injuries and epilepsy, which may exacerbate damage to the brain. On the other hand, people with cognitive impairment, particularly where there is disinhibition as in fronto-temporal dementia (📖 Chapter 15), may present to alcohol treatment services when the normal social controls on their drinking are affected by their illness.

Korsakoff's syndrome

In this condition there is a profound and irreversible inability to lay down new memories. People with this disorder have intact long-term memories up to a specific time, but can remember nothing thereafter. They are able to retain new information for a few minutes, but not for any longer (Chapter 6 p. 67). Many people with Korsakoff's syndrome make up stories to cover up their deficits (confabulation). There are often other impairments, with slowed cognition and reduced motivation, and sometimes other neurological signs, such as cerebellar ataxia or peripheral neuropathy.

Reversible dementia

Although the definition in Box 1.1 does not rule out the possibility of the disorder being reversible, in practice disease processes that cause dementia almost never remit completely. It is sometimes suggested that intra-cranial space occupying lesions (tumours and subdural haematomas), hypothyroidism, or vitamin deficiencies can produce a dementia syndrome, but the symptoms in these illnesses are usually closer to those typical of delirium (📖 Chapter 3) than to those of dementia. Metabolic disturbances are often incidental findings rather than the cause of dementia. It is unusual for cognitive or behavioural symptoms to resolve after laboratory values return to normal. However, it is always worthwhile trying to improve the general health of people with dementia as much as possible to promote or maintain quality of life.

Normal pressure hydrocephalus

In this rare disorder, difficult to diagnose (or exclude), there is impairment in the drainage of cerebrospinal fluid (CSF), which accumulates in the cerebral ventricles, although CSF pressure is not grossly raised. Insertion of a shunt to drain CSF can lead to dramatic clinical improvement.

Key symptoms
- Insidious memory impairment.
- Ataxic gait.
- Urinary incontinence—more severe than would be expected from the degree of cognitive impairment.

Supportive features
- Psychomotor retardation or apathy.
- History of meningitis, head injury or subarachnoid haemorrhage.
- CT scan appearances showing widening of the cerebral ventricles with periventricular changes but without much atrophy of the gyri.

Treatment
- Refer to a neurologist for diagnostic lumbar puncture.
- If there is improvement (judged by measured cognitive performance, timed walking and qualitative gait assessment) when about 30 ml of CSF is removed then surgical insertion of a shunt may be helpful.

Space occupying lesions

Cognitive impairment is the commonest psychological symptom of an intra-cranial space occupying lesion. Most commonly there are features of focal damage rather than generalized dementia. Apart from memory loss, slowed thinking, and slow and incoherent speech, poor judgement or perseveration are characteristic. Slowly growing tumours (especially neoplasms of the non-dominant temporal lobe) rarely cause any psychological symptoms.

Metastases are the most likely cerebral tumours to cause neuropsychiatric symptoms, and meningiomas are less likely to cause dementia than gliomas.

Symptoms that may indicate the presence of a tumour include:
- Irritability.
- Depression.
- Apathy.
- Euphoria.

nat is not dementia

epression

Depression is very common among elderly people, and depression and dementia often co-exist. About 20% of people with dementia have comorbid depression.

Around 30% of general hospital inpatients and 12% of the general population over 65 will have depression according to the criteria in Box 1.5. Most antidepressants are safe and well-tolerated, and many older people are now receiving prescriptions for antidepressants.

People with depression have difficulty in concentrating on external events because of their preoccupation with their inner feelings of lack of hope. They often perform badly on tests of cognitive function and the possibility of organic brain disease can be raised. Cognitive problems other than impairment of memory and concentration are not part of depression, so problems in language, drawing and executive function make a diagnosis of dementia probable.

Screening tests such as Hospital Anxiety and Depression Scale or Geriatric Depression Scale may be helpful in assessing depression and anxiety. The Cornell Scale for Depression in Dementia, which is completed by an informant, is useful in more severe dementia (📖 Chapter 13 p. 330).

Serious depression (bad enough to cause attention and memory problems) is likely to be obvious. Diurnal variation, with problems most severe in the early morning, improving as the day goes on, is characteristic of depression, but is not found in dementia.

'Depressive pseudo-dementia' is a term sometimes used for people whose cognitive impairment is attributed to depression. On follow-up, most of these people go on to develop unequivocal dementia.

Treatment of depression

The recommended first line treatment of mild depression is to increase physical activity—not always feasible in frail older people.

For moderate depression medication can be tried—citalopram and trazodone are good first line choices.

Box 1.5 Symptoms of depression

- Persistent sadness or low mood; and/or
- Loss of interests or pleasure.
- Fatigue or low energy.

Associated symptoms:
  - change in appetite or weight
  - change in sleep pattern
  - poor concentration
  - feelings of guilt or worthlessness
  - hypochondriacal beliefs
  - suicidal ideas
  - agitation or slowing of movement.

Box 1.6 Symptoms of anxiety

- Autonomic:
  - palpitations
  - sweating
  - tremor
  - dry mouth.
- Chest and abdominal symptoms:
  - difficulty breathing
  - feeling of choking, chest pain or discomfort
  - nausea or abdominal distress.
- Mental symptoms:
  - feelings of unreality
  - fear of losing control
  - fear of dying.
- General:
  - feeling dizzy or faint
  - hot flushes or shivering
  - numbness or tingling
  - muscle tension
  - restlessness
  - lump in throat
  - mind going blank
  - persistent irritability
  - difficulty getting to sleep because of worrying.

- Citalopram: start at 10 mg daily (larger doses may cause GI disturbance and exacerbate appetite loss, which is common in depression). Most people with depression will need 20–30 mg daily.
- Trazodone: start with 50–100 mg at bedtime, although it can be given in divided doses during the day if agitation is a problem. Older people are likely to respond to 50–150 mg daily but the dose can be increased up to 300 mg/day if necessary. Apart from sedation, adverse effects are unusual.

In resistant cases or where anxiety and sleep disturbance is prominent, mirtazapine (15–30 mg at night) may be helpful.

Severe cases of depression, particularly where there are thoughts of suicide, should be referred to a psychiatrist.

Psychological therapies such as cognitive behaviour therapy (CBT) or interpersonal psychotherapy are effective for mild to moderate depression, but skilled practitioners who can deliver these treatments to older people are in short supply and waiting lists may be long.

Anxiety

It is difficult to draw a clear dividing line between depression and anxiety. About 3% of older people in the community suffer from anxiety; in general hospitals the figure is approximately 8%. The key symptom of anxiety is of autonomic arousal (Box 1.6).

Anxiety is often subdivided into three syndromes:

- Panic disorder.
- Generalized anxiety disorder.
- Phobic anxiety—where there is a particular fear, such as needles, face masks, spiders etc., or of social situations.

In extreme cases anxiety may lead to loss of capacity to make informed decisions on treatment, but it will almost never cause confusion. The most effective treatment for anxiety disorders is cognitive behavioural therapy. A trial of an SSRI antidepressant is usually justified whilst awaiting psychological therapy. An acute onset of anxiety and confusion should always raise the possibility of delirium.

Mania

Mania is a rare disorder in the age group at risk of dementia and delirium, but it can occur as a result of acute physical disorders such as stroke. The key symptoms are given in Box 1.7. Patients with mania need to be referred to a psychiatrist for specialist management. It is important to differentiate between mania and the disinhibition and grandiosity found in fronto-temporal dementia (📖 Chapter 15).

Paranoid psychosis

Paranoid symptoms may be present in dementia, especially DLB. They also occur in delirium and depression. True paranoid psychosis is rare but worth diagnosing as it may respond well to medication. Cognitive testing shows intact memory and intellect.

Typical paranoid symptoms include:

- Persecution by neighbours or family.
- Control by external agencies.

- Preoccupation with bizarre sexual practices.
- Auditory hallucinations are sometimes present, and there is often an association with deafness and tinnitus.
- Visual hallucinations are highly suggestive of DLB.

Sometimes persecutory disorders in older people may be a result of long standing schizophrenia.

Antipsychotic medication is often dramatically effective, but always consider the possibility of DLB (as people with DLB are at risk of severe extrapyramidal side effects, even with atypical antipsychotics). People with paranoid psychosis rarely develop insight into the psychological origin of their symptoms and so it is often difficult to persuade them to persevere with medication, particularly if side effects occur. There is no evidence that people who do not have dementia are at increased risk of cerebrovascular disease as a result of taking antipsychotic medication.

Box 1.7 Symptoms of mania

- Elevation of mood or irritability.
- Increased activity, restlessness.
- Increased talkativeness.
- Flight of ideas, feeling thoughts racing.
- Increased self esteem.
- Impaired concentration, distractibility.
- Decreased need for sleep.
- Increased sexual energy.
- Overspending, other reckless behaviour.

ummary

1. Dementia is a condition of progressive, global, cognitive impairment.
2. The most common causes are Alzheimer's disease, vascular dementia and dementia with Lewy bodies.
3. Delirium and functional psychiatric illnesses such as anxiety and depression also need to be considered as possible causes of impaired memory and thinking.

Chapter 2

Assessment

Introduction

A characteristic feature of illness in old age is non-specificity of presentation. 'Confusion' (along with the other 'geriatric giants' of immobility, falls and incontinence) may be the result of many different disease processes.

The presentation of cognitive disorders is further complicated by:
- Lack of insight, so that problems presented to health care professionals are diverse and may be denied by the patient.
- Difficulty in ascertaining information necessary for diagnosis, because of cognitive impairment, other communication problems (e.g. deafness, language), or physical illness.
- Misinterpretation of signs and symptoms by families and carers, and many health professionals, or ignorance of their significance.
- Symptoms or their severity may be denied by families, or compensated for as part of normal social reciprocity (e.g. a son or daughter doing the shopping or paying the bills).

This also means that a variety of professionals may be the first point of contact. All need skills in recognizing and assessing cognitive impairment, and a knowledge of where to direct patients and their families for appropriate further help. Professional groups include:
- General practitioners.
- Community nurses.
- Hospital doctors, in any adult specialty.
- Hospital nurses, in Accident and Emergency departments, admissions wards, or any adult inpatient or outpatient setting.
- Social workers.
- Occupational therapists and physiotherapists (community and hospital).
- Specialist nurses, such as continence advisors, diabetic nurses or respiratory nurses.
- Managers and workers in care homes or day centres.
- Voluntary sector services.

Presenting problems

We hope that our first encounter with a confused patient will occur in the best circumstances: the patient relaxed and confident in familiar surroundings and accompanied by a reliable informant.

However, the initial contact often takes place in difficult surroundings: an accident unit, a medical ward, or a hospital clinic. Whatever the circumstances it will be possible to make some sort of diagnostic assessment.

Dementia should only be diagnosed after a comprehensive assessment. This should include:

- History from the patient and an informant.
- Physical and mental state examination.
- A review of medication.
- Any necessary investigations.

It is important to interpret the results of any assessment in the light of the person's educational and employment background, and their physical health, eyesight, and hearing.

Memory loss, severe misjudgement or bizarre behaviour are easy enough clues that there may be a problem with cognition. But cognitive problems sometimes 'emerge' rather than 'present'; for example, unexpected difficulty in basic daily activities after recovery from an acute illness, or failure to progress in rehabilitation. In retrospect, it may become clear that problems have been present for some months previously.

Presentations include:

- 'Confusion'—often referred to in requests for help from families or in referrals between professionals, but it is a vague term and needs further clarification.
- Memory loss, forgetfulness, or related behaviours such as repetitiveness, may be reported by the patient or relatives.
- Functional decline—work performance, not coping, increasing requirements for help.
- Unexpected, inappropriate, unacceptable or bizarre behaviours—wandering, agitation, aggression, hoarding, disrobing; perhaps leading to a crisis, such as getting lost or making accusations against or hitting a family member.
- Misjudgement—sometimes of monumental proportions, such as trying to walk miles or repair the television set unaided.
- 'Decompensation':
  - Anything that disrupts routine and familiarity (moving house, a holiday, going into hospital) may lead to disproportionate functional decline—an inability to cope.
  - Sudden loss of a carer (death of a spouse, son or daughter on holiday).
- Incidental (during a presentation for another illness). Ward or care home staff may notice that something is not quite right, or that expected progress is not being made. But a cursory assessment (social niceties on a ward round) may fail to recognize the existence or extent of cognitive problems.

The job of the health care professional is to identify the problems and reach an explanation. This can be surprisingly difficult for the inexperienced, especially if a convincing social facade is retained. You need to think broadly and laterally, know what to expect, and overcome embarrassment.

In some cases a single diagnosis, or group of diagnoses, may be sufficient. However, more useful is the idea of 'formulation'—an explanation in terms of diagnosis, comorbidity, and social and psychological elements, of how a person's problems arose.

This implies collecting a wide variety of information on symptoms, problems, comorbidities, abilities and disabilities, human and material resources, wants and preferences, and lifestyle. Always consider the possibility of cognitive decline when problems are vague, non-specific, or don't quite add up.

'Confusion'

Confusion is a vague and non-specific term. The *Concise Oxford Dictionary* defines it as 'throwing into disorder, mixing up in the mind, perplexed'. It implies abnormal thinking, lacking clarity or coherence, or the behavioural consequences of irrational or illogical thought.

Confusion may indicate a cognitive impairment. But it may also reflect other things that must be distinguished:

- Psychosis—characterized by abnormality of perception (visual, auditory or tactile hallucinations) or delusions (abnormal beliefs).
- Depression—mood disorder with sadness, pessimism, hopelessness, slowness, or agitation.
- Mania—a disorder of affect, with over-arousal, over-activity, grandiose or over-optimistic thought, and a lack of insight and judgement.
- Anxiety—a state of worry or fearfulness, with psychological and somatic elements (including palpitation, hyperventilation, dry mouth, and/or abdominal discomfort).
- Dysphasia—a disorder of language, commonly seen after a stroke. Speech may be impossible, words may be jumbled or used wrongly, or understanding may be impaired.
- Eccentricity, in some cases leading to apparent neglect of customary tidiness or hygiene (Diogenes' syndrome).

Cognitive impairment

There are three main syndromes of cognitive impairment:

- Delirium.
- Learning disability (low intellect, intellectual impairment, 'mental handicap').
- Dementia.

Distinguishing these is a key task. It is made all the more difficult because relatives and many health professionals are ignorant of the distinctions and implications, and it is only when an experienced practitioner is involved that the explanation emerges. Even then it may be couched with uncertainty.

The distinction is important because delirium is usually reversible, often indicates severe physical illness, and has a high mortality. Unless it is recognized, management will be wrong, treatment for physical illness not instituted, and important decisions (for example about moving into a care home) may be taken on the basis of false presumptions. Opportunities for improvement will be missed and future options limited.

Delirium (📖 Chapter 3)
Delirium is a disorder of:
- Abnormal cognition (i.e. 'confusion').
- Abnormal attention and arousal (agitation, lethargy, or drowsiness; altered sleep-wake cycle).

That is:
- Usually fluctuating (generally over hours; a single clinical assessment will not make the diagnosis so ask the relatives or nurses).
- Acute onset (although it is ten times commoner in people with pre-existing dementia).
- Due to an identifiable physical cause (but identifying it can be difficult).
- Reversible with treatment of the physical disease (may be slower than you expect—2 to 4 weeks or more).
- Often (or usually) missed by medical doctors (people are generally inattentive and 'under the weather' in moderate to severe illness, and applying the tests can be difficult).

There may also be:
- Disordered thinking.
- Incoherence, such as rambling or irrelevant conversation, illogical flow of ideas, or unpredictable switching from subject to subject.
- Misperceptions and hallucinations—usually visual and frightening.
- Paranoia.

The main alternative diagnoses are:
- Dementia with Lewy bodies (also characterized by confusion, fluctuation and hallucinations, almost always with signs of Parkinsonism. Beware extrapyramidal side effects of antipsychotic drugs).
- Progression of vascular dementia (the steps of a 'stepwise decline' include a sudden deterioration).
- Decompensation of pre-existing dementia:
  - disorientation, bewilderment, fear, or agitation in a strange environment (e.g. new day centre or hospital)
  - a behavioural crisis (due to poor memory or insight, misjudgement, or disinhibition).
- Pure disorders of alertness:
  - drowsiness due to neurological disease (raised intra-cranial pressure, infections, stroke, or tumours)
  - sedation due to drugs.
- Disorders of communication (dysphasia, deafness).
- Post-ictal confusion.
- Other primary psychiatric disorders: depression, mania, functional psychosis, schizophrenia.
- Others: thiamine deficiency, head injury, transient global amnesia (TGA).

Learning disability

This implies a congenital or acquired abnormality of cognitive and learni ability, present from childhood. It is non-progressive in terms of neuro-logical damage, but, with both childhood development and under the influence of social and physical environmental factors, functional and behavioural manifestations may vary over time. Genetic, intrauterine, birth injury, and early life brain injury (traumatic, toxic or infective) are all pos-sible causes. In addition, further acquired deterioration in the form of a superadded dementia may develop in mid- or older-adult life.

Intelligence (and other cognitive functions) varies between individuals, and forms a spectrum across the whole population. People with low intel-ligence (sometimes called 'borderline learning disabled') who have not been formally diagnosed with an intellectual disability may cause diag-nostic difficulty if illness or disability in older age cause difficulty coping with functional tasks that have previously been accommodated.

Dementia (📖 Chapter 1)

Dementia is a progressive disorder with global impairment of cognitive functions (although it is common that some are affected more than others, at least initially).

Common to all dementias are:
- Cognitive decline: in memory, orientation, concentration, intellect, insight, executive function (decision-making, judgement), and, later, language, praxis (ability to do purposeful activity), and visuo-spatial awareness.
- Functional impairment: initially instrumental activities of daily living (e.g. using things, driving, managing finances, going on the bus, cooking), and then more basic functions.
- Behavioural change: passivity, sleep disturbance, anxiety, bewilderment, frustration, agitation, and wandering.

The process of assessment and diagnosis

To make a diagnosis, consider history—including third party history—mental state examination, physical examination, tests of cognitive function, descriptions of function at home or on a ward, investigations, and follow-up.

(i) The history—from patient and carer

It is generally appropriate to start by trying to take a history from the patient. Box 2.1 offers suggestions about how to go about this. But you cannot diagnose dementia, nor differentiate it from delirium, without a third party history.

It doesn't matter whether you speak to the informant before or after you see the patient, but try to devote your full attention to the patient whilst you're with them and discourage carers from interrupting when you're speaking to the patient. It can be helpful to have carers present; the presence of familiar figures may be reassuring. The carers will know which aspects of the patient's account may need amendment. They may be surprised to discover what the patient is capable of if given the opportunity.

What is more important is to have the opportunity to speak to the carers without the patient present. Think of it as 'clerking the relatives'. Identifying and characterizing prior cognitive function is key. They may also wish to pass on information that would be upsetting if discussed in the presence of the patient. Even if there is clear evidence of impairment, carers often wish to ensure that you understand what they are experiencing, especially where there is fluctuation in the condition. If there has been a sudden change, delirium or a delirium mimic is likely.

Remember that early forgetfulness, lapses in judgement, or personality changes may not be recognized as such, or may be ignored, suppressed or compensated for (by family members taking on more mentally difficult tasks). Your third party history-taking will have to probe—who does the bills, the shopping; what does the patient do to occupy their time? Inability to do mentally taxing tasks may only become apparent when a spouse becomes ill or dies.

Impairment of recent memory is often dismissed by patients and families, frequently as part of normal ageing. Indeed in quantitative terms there is no clear distinction between 'normal' and 'abnormal' ageing. Measurements of cognitive function lie on a continuum. It is when the problems stretch across multiple domains, are clearly progressive, and interfere with social function, without an alternative explanation, that dementia is diagnosable.

Note:
- What led the patient to present to medical attention?
- Duration, fluctuation or progression of symptoms. (When did you first notice a problem? When was he or she last normal? How were things last Christmas? Last summer?)
- Forgetfulness, repetitiveness.
- Misplacing or losing things (and consequent accusations of theft).

- Safety concerns such as leaving the gas on, burning out pans, getting lost, dealing with strangers, hazardous driving.
- Reasoning and judgement.
- Change in personality and behaviour.
- Night-time disturbance (sleep reversal).
- Loss of hygiene and house sense (living in squalor).
- Continence.
- Falls.
- Insight.

Remember that others may have useful information. Consider phoning the family doctor, or social care providers (home care, or wardens of assisted living facilities). The drug history is important, especially recent changes, and will often not be reliably given by the patient. Was mental state or physical function recorded during a previous hospital admission?

Box 2.1 Taking a history from a patient

- Stay calm, friendly, natural and confident.
- Introduce yourself, speak simply. Explain why you're there.
- Find out what the patient likes to be called. Older people may feel threatened if you use their first name; if you are going to use a fore-name then make sure it's the right one. Mary Jane Evans may always be called Jane by her friends and family; 'The only time I'm ever called Mary is at the hospital.'
- Take a careful note of the patient's behaviour and appearance.
- Listen to what the patient has to say. If their speech seems garbled, write down some of their utterances and try to make sense of them later. Don't diagnose dysphasia without including examples.
- If they're happy to talk, join them in some general conversation to establish a good relationship. It is easier to assess the form of speech in social interaction than when asking questions to establish informa-tion. If they have questions, answer them honestly.
- Find out what the patient sees as the problem and take this seriously; people with dementia may see their main difficulty as something other than their memory and may rapidly lose patience if you ignore the problems that trouble them.
- If it's not mentioned spontaneously, ask if they are at all forgetful.
- Start with basic questions about orientation to person and place. If there are difficulties here, find out how memory problems are causing difficulty.
- Establish the current home situation as the patient sees it. It is often helpful to run through the course of a typical day with the patient.
- Fill in background:
  - members of the family
  - place of origin, education and occupation (in order to have some idea of the pre-morbid level of cognitive functioning)
  - previous medical history.
- Attempt more specific assessment of cognitive function e.g. MMSE.
- Ask about mood, anxieties and preoccupations.
- Establishing the presence of psychotic symptoms can often be dif-ficult; examples of common symptoms are in the text sections *Abnormal beliefs* and *Abnormal perceptions* (📖 p. 35).

(ii) Examine the mental state (rudiments for non-psychiatrists)

Examination is a combination of observation and questioning. This may have to be subtle or may be difficult if the patient is suspicious or unco-operative.

The objective is to characterize cognitive deficits and exclude depression, psychosis or other psychiatric diagnoses (see Box 2.2).

Note:

- Appearance—grooming, dress, distress.
- Behaviour—agitation, apathy, co-operation, eye contact.
- Cognition:
  - alertness
  - orientation (person, place, time)
  - concentration
  - memory—registration and short-term recall
  - intellect
  - abstract thought and decision-making.
- Speech—amount, volume, rate—beware aphasia, and specifically test for it (understanding motor commands, fluency in spontaneous conversation or picture description, naming, sequences, yes/no).
- Mood, objective and subjective.
- Thoughts, including delusions.
- Hallucinations.
- Insight.

Mood

In psychiatric terminology, 'mood' refers to the person's inner, subjective feelings (their objective outward appearance is the 'affect'). People with depression don't always complain of feeling sad. Look out also for persistent negative ideas—of being a being a burden, not deserving other people's efforts, or of lack of motivation. If depressive symptoms are present, ask explicitly about thoughts of self-harm.

It is often difficult to differentiate rational beliefs about difficult life situations from depressive cognitions; the most useful test is to establish whether the person is able to experience some enjoyment. Inability to cheer up in normally rewarding situations (anhedonia) is a reliable sign of depression. Mood rating scales (Chapter 13) are worth considering, if only as a general checklist for possible symptoms. The Geriatric Depression Scale or the Hospital Anxiety and Depression Scale are useful for older people who may also have physical health problems. The Cornell Scale can be used to elicit symptoms of depression from an informant for a person with dementia.

Box 2.2 Mental state examination

- Appearance and behaviour:
  - anxious or relaxed?
  - happy or sad?
  - smart or scruffy?
  - clean or dirty?
- Speech:
  - rate, rhythm and volume of speech
  - structure of speech—is it grammatical?
  - does it make sense?
  - problems finding words?
  - making up words?
- Mood.
- Abnormal beliefs (delusions):
  - this man isn't my husband
  - people are moving things at home
  - this isn't my home
  - strangers are coming into my home.
- Abnormal perceptions (hallucinations):
  - seeing strangers around the home
  - seeing faces or insects on furnishings
  - hearing singing
  - hearing people talking.
- Cognition.
- Insight.
- Personality—present and previous.

Abnormal beliefs

Many firmly held false beliefs in people with dementia are the direct result of memory impairment. Some people with dementia lack insight about their poor recollection of where they left their purse, keys, spectacles etc. and may think that others have moved them; if no one else is around they may believe that burglars have broken in to the house to steal them. Other common delusions include not recognizing one's spouse or one's home—which may result from imagining that they are much younger. Believing that one is being kept a prisoner may also be easy to understand. Delusions that are not comprehensible in the light of cognitive impairment may also occur; only this type of false belief is likely to respond well to treatment with antipsychotic medication.

Abnormal perceptions

Auditory hallucinations are most commonly the result of functional psychoses, such as schizophrenia or severe depression, although they may occur in DLB. People with tinnitus may also believe that they can hear voices in the background. Visual hallucinations frequently occur in DLB, and sometimes in AD. They often involve seeing strangers in one's home, they are especially common in people with poor eyesight, and they are most frequent where lighting conditions lead to ambiguous shadows. Visual hallucinations are not always unwelcome; lonely elderly people may delight in watching little people dancing around their gardens or children eating at their tables.

(iii) Physical examination

A full physical examination is required, including a thorough and competent neurological examination.

Often the most relevant physical signs can be deduced from simply observing the patient. Watch their gait for signs of weakness, unsteadiness, and pain. Look at their facial expression, pupils and mouth. Are there any abnormal movements present?

Note alertness and any fluctuation during the examination. Look for extrapyramidal signs (increased limb tone, tremor, bradykinesia) and any involuntary movements (dyskinesias in Parkinson's disease, chorea in Huntingdon's disease, myoclonus in Creutzfeldt-Jakob disease, tremor or flap (asterixis) in metabolic encephalopathy). Look for pyramidal motor signs (weakness, increased tone, brisk reflexes and upgoing plantars).

In the absence of suggestive history (focal onset seizures, raised intracranial pressure), a normal neurological examination makes a structural brain lesion unlikely.

General physical examination is required to seek causes of delirium and define comorbidities. Arthritis, in particular, is very common and often poorly documented.

(iv) Tests of cognitive function

Having one's memory tested can be a shaming and distressing experience. Many people feel profoundly embarrassed at being unable to answer simple questions. Some people are proficient at avoiding direct responses; they try to get others to speak for them or attempt to persuade the questioner to give a clue as to the correct response. Often the practitioner can ense the distress that the impaired person is trying to avoid, but at the end of the day it is necessary to establish the diagnosis. This can only be done by confirming the level of cognitive function. You can do this 'free-style', as part of the mental state examination, or use a structured questionnaire (☐ Chapter 13 p. 323–5).

The Folstein Mini-Mental State Examination (MMSE) is the standard. It is much more sophisticated than the 10-point Hodkinson Abbreviated Mental Test score (AMT). It is not hard to memorize and is very widely used and understood (although many would argue technically imperfect). It includes:

- Orientation to time (5 points).
- Orientation to place (5 points).
- Registration of three objects (3 points).
- 'world' backwards, or the first five serial sevens (5 points).
- Three objects recall (3 points).
- Writing a sentence (1 point).
- Three stage command (3 points).
- Naming two objects (2 points).
- Repeating 'no ifs, ands, or buts' (1 point).
- Copying intersecting pentagons (1 point).
- Reading and performing 'close your eyes' (1 point).

There are well-validated alternatives to the MMSE, which may be especially useful in primary care. These include the 6-item Cognitive Impairment Test (6-CIT) and the 7-minute screen.

The AMT is convenient as a screening tool in hurried and difficult settings such as Emergency Departments or Medical Admission wards. But it is no more than that, a screening tool, which will require proper follow-up if suggestive of a problem. Other disciplines (such as occupational therapy) commonly use different assessment tools (e.g. MEAMS).

It is useful to be able to assess executive function using the trail making test (tracing out a path between numbered points) and a test of verbal fluency (timed naming of animals, or words beginning with a particular letter). The Cognitive Estimates test can give an idea about grandiosity.

In cases of doubt or particular need, more extensive formal neuropsychological testing batteries can be used.

(v) Home or ward reports and observation—assessment of behaviour and activities of daily living

Partly this flows from the history. But once care services are involved over a period of time, there is the opportunity to make objective observations of behaviour and function.

Assessment can be misleading in a pressurized or unfamiliar environment (such as a clinic), or if a doctor visiting at home induces anxiety or brings out 'best behaviour'. So may a brief (20–30 minutes) home assessment visit as part of discharge planning after a hospital stay. Observations of day to day functioning in occupation, nursing and therapy activities may be better.

This can include level periods of drowsiness or hyperactivity, fluctuations over time, activities of daily living, self-management of medication, safety awareness, judgement and decision-making, wandering, shouting or disturbed behaviour, and night-time problems. More complex functions like kitchen use and safety can be assessed, but may require several sessions, as the environment will be unfamiliar.

Ultimately a 'trial of discharge' from hospital can be seen as a period of observation.

(vi) Physical investigations

In primary care

These (Table 2.1) mainly screen for potential causes of delirium and comorbidities, rather than causes of dementia *per se*.

Routine haematology helps to exclude concomitant medical illness. Vitamin B12 and folate levels are customarily checked; however, there is little evidence that treating low levels of haematinics improves cognitive performance.

Biochemical tests include testing for levels of electrolytes, calcium, and glucose, and for thyroid, renal, and liver function. By the time dementia has developed there is not much evidence that correcting hypothyroidism or reducing elevated plasma glucose (or cholesterol) makes much difference to the long-term outcome, but optimizing physical health is a good general principle. C-reactive protein (CRP) and erythrocyte sedimentation rate (ESR) are non-specific markers of disease, especially infection. An abnormal CRP test should prompt further investigation in the patient who appears unwell but lacks clear-cut signs or symptoms of disease.

An ECG should be done where clinically indicated. It is a non-invasive and generally helpful test. Cholinesterase inhibitors and antipsychotic drugs can potentially cause cardiac problems and having a baseline ECG can be useful.

Table 2.1 Investigation in primary care

Investigation	Tests
Haematology	Full blood count and ESR or CRP
	B12 and folate
Biochemistry	Urea, creatinine, electrolytes (U + E), calcium
	Liver function tests
	Thyroid function tests
	Blood glucose
	Lipids
Urinalysis and culture	
ECG	

Investigation by specialist teams

Serological testing

Syphilis and AIDS are rare causes of dementia in developed countries. There is no need to screen routinely for evidence of infection. Discuss early with a neurologist or microbiologist which tests are likely to be most useful if these are suspected.

If the ESR or CRP are raised, autoimmune causes of dementia such as SLE are a possibility. Investigate further with anti-nuclear antibody and other auto-antibodies. If CRP or ESR are consistently raised when the patient is confused and there is no indication of infection, some form of 'steroid sensitive disease' is a possibility. These are often associated with a low lymphocyte count. Detailed investigation may not reveal a cause, although an LP during a period of confusion may show inflammatory markers, suggesting a cerebral vasculitis. A trial of prednisolone 30 mg/day is worthwhile.

Chest X-ray (CXR)

Only do this where there is a clinical indication. Auscultation is notoriously unreliable for diagnosis of chest infections in older people; increased respiratory rate may be a more valuable pointer.

EEG

An EEG is not normally recommended in the investigation of Alzheimer's disease. However, a normal EEG makes a diagnosis of delirium unlikely. The EEG may be markedly abnormal in even mild DLB. The combination of normal structural imaging and abnormal EEG is highly suggestive of DLB (📖 Box 1.4, p. 11). There may be characteristic EEG appearances (triphasic waves) in people with classical CJD. The EEG is also helpful in assessing seizure disorders in dementia.

Diagnostic imaging

Lay people (and doctors) place great faith in scans, and some form of imaging is recommended by NICE. In practice the CT scan has limited value; it is helpful mostly for excluding significant focal lesions of brain tissue—stroke, haematoma, or tumour—and normal pressure hydrocephalus.

Indications for urgent CT scan:
- Rapid deterioration.
- Unexplained focal neurological signs or symptoms.
- Head injury.
- Early ataxia or urinary incontinence.

In the diagnosis of early onset dementia, MRI imaging is more useful. It allows for a better assessment of temporal lobe anatomy, and this is particularly helpful if fronto-temporal dementia is suspected. Marked atrophy of the medial temporal lobes is nearly always due to Alzheimer's disease.

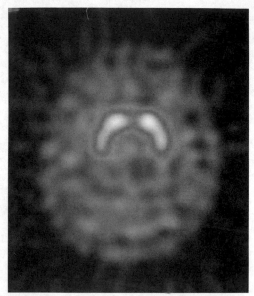

Fig. 2.1 Normal appearance of DaTSCAN®. See also Plate 1, Plate Section.

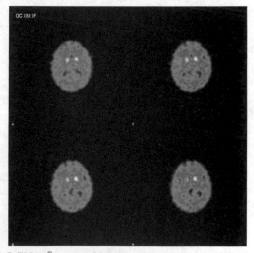

Fig. 2.2 DaTSCAN® in a case of dementia with Lewy bodies, showing reduced uptake of isotope into the caudate nuclei. See also Plate 2, Plate section (Courtesy of GE Healthcare).

Single photon emission computed tomography (SPECT) is sometimes helpful in sorting out different causes of dementia. The ligand exametazine demonstrates cerebral blood flow and can be helpful in separating Alzheimer's, fronto-temporal and vascular dementia, so long as a radiologist with experience in interpreting SPECT scans is available. exametazine-SPECT cannot be used to investigate people with learning disabilities, who have lifelong changes on SPECT scans resembling those found in Alzheimer's disease.

Ioflupane (*DaTSCAN*®) is a ligand that binds to dopamine receptors (Fig. 2.1). The comma-shaped appearance of the basal ganglia becomes more elliptical in people with DLB or Parkinson's disease dementia (Fig. 2.2). Dementia with Lewy bodies is usually relatively easy to recognize clinically, but in cases of doubt ioflupane SPECT can be valuable.

Lumbar puncture
CSF examination is not helpful in the diagnosis of commonly encountered forms of dementia. When it is necessary it is best left to a specialist neurologist (as a bloody tap may make the sample useless). It is indicated in the diagnosis of intra-cranial infection, cerebral vasculitis, and Creutzfeldt-Jakob disease.

Diagnosis of subtypes (📖 Chapters 1 and 15)

This is a job for a specialist who is familiar with agreed international criteria for Alzheimer's disease, vascular dementia, dementia with Lewy bodies, and fronto-temporal dementia.

It is not clear what benefit there is in trying to split Alzheimer's disease and vascular dementia. Most people with dementia will have some elements of both disorders present, they all need to have their vascular risk factors considered, and most deserve a trial with a cholinesterase inhibitor. Identifying dementia with Lewy bodies has clear value in terms of management (e.g. avoidance of antipsychotic drugs) and explanation of fluctuation and other sometimes bewildering symptoms.

Cognitive impairment in people with learning disability
(📖 Chapters 14)

If a person with a learning disability is found to be functioning less well than previously it is important to exclude causes such as musculo-skeletal problems, deafness, or poor sight. Thyroid disease and cardiovascular disorders are also frequently found. Stressful life events and mental disorders such as anxiety, depression, and delirium may also be responsible. Only after considering these factors is it worthwhile asking a clinical psychologist to undertake tests for assessing cognitive function in learning disability.

Incidental or comorbid dementia

Dementia is often not diagnosed, but becomes apparent when a related or separate problem arises. Emergency or elective surgical admissions are a time of particular risk. There is a break with the familiar environment and routine (decompensation), the possibility of disease-related or post-operative delirium, and care procedures that may be misunderstood or seen as threatening (such as cannula insertion or urethral catheterization). Much the same also holds for admissions to medical or other wards.

Dementia may also become apparent when a care home placement is arranged. The 'social response' to non-specific failure to cope may be to provide substitute care, and once there it becomes apparent that cognitive problems explain or contribute to the failure to cope.

Screening and early diagnosis

Given the difficulties in recognizing cognitive impairment before a crisis arises, should we screen everyone (perhaps over a certain age) using a tool such as the MMSE?

In some settings this is sensible—such as acute geriatric or medical admissions, or after a stroke. Sometimes it will be useful to have a baseline against which future changes may be compared (e.g. on care home admission). But applying these tests universally is time-consuming, will carry a burden of false positive results (which may cause anxiety, require further assessment, and subsequent reassurance), and may be thought demeaning by patients. If staff are alert and well-trained, screening should not always be necessary.

Unfortunately in many settings this is not the case, and new junior staff will always need to be accommodated. Even the most experienced staff can be caught out. If patients object to necessary testing, items can be embedded in a more general conversation. But most do not mind doing a 'memory test'. More experienced practitioners may choose to be selective in whom they test, but should always hold a low threshold for formal cognitive testing.

Abnormal scores on screening tests do not make a diagnosis of dementia; problems in daily living as a result of impaired cognition are also required. Sometimes all that can be done is to make a diagnosis of mild cognitive impairment (📖 Chapter 1 p. 13) and keep things under regular review.

Don't get it wrong

Be careful not to diagnose dementia when the history really does not support it. Labels carelessly written in the notes sometimes stick.

Sharing the diagnosis

People vary enormously in their wish to have a diagnosis given to them. Gentle questioning at an early stage will help to ascertain what people can, and want to, be told. For some the terms 'Alzheimer's disease' or 'dementia' are as terrifying as 'cancer', but they are not distressed to be told that they have memory impairment that is related to the ageing process. Some people have experience of dealing with people with advanced dementia and are petrified by the thought of becoming the helpless resident of a nursing home.

It is important to make it clear that the condition is not curable but may respond to appropriate treatment (including medication) in the short term. It is ultimately going to get worse and may cause disability requiring considerable levels of support. Nearly everybody has a pretty shrewd idea of what is going on before they reach secondary care services. Telling falsehoods to patients is never justified but it is often charitable to give people a chance to adapt to the truth. Depression is common in the early stages of dementia, but it does not seem to be any more common amongst people who have been told their diagnosis.

Planning for the future

Once a diagnosis of dementia is confirmed, planning for the future needs to be considered (📖 Chapter 12).
- Should treatment with an acetyl cholinesterase inhibitor (AChEI) be started? (📖 Chapter 6 p. 140)
- Can driving continue? (📖 Chapter 5 p. 132)
- Are plans in place to make decisions in the event of future incapacity? (📖 Chapter 11)
  - power of attorney
  - advanced refusal of treatment
  - has the patient made a will?
- Do the family or friends need education or support? (📖 Chapter 5 p. 124)
- Should a move to sheltered housing be considered?

Copying doctors' letters to patients

It is now a common practice in the UK, encouraged by the government, to send copies of clinic letters from hospital specialists to general practitioners to the patient.

Patients generally appreciate this, and it can be a useful way of educating patients about their conditions. However, there are ethical issues about this practice where the person about whom the letter is written may not be able to fully understand its contents, even if it is drafted in simple language. Often a definitive diagnosis is not made at the initial clinic appointment and it is generally not appropriate to send a patient a letter in which there is speculation about diagnosis. It is also possible for letters to be picked up by people from whom the subject would wish to withhold confidential clinical information.

Surveys have shown that patients and their families want clear verbal information about the diagnosis and its implications, and the treatment and support they can expect. Relatives and carers are usually more enthusiastic about receiving written information on diagnosis and investigation than the person with suspected cognitive impairment. Sometimes information or instructions can be addressed, out of courtesy, to the GP (or patient) whilst primarily being aimed at carers. If the patient is happy for written information to be passed on, and has the capacity to consent to the letter being sent to a carer (including the staff of care homes), then there is no reason why this should not happen.

Holders of registered welfare powers of attorney are also entitled to receive copies of letters.

Summary

1. Confusion may be due to dementia, delirium or something else entirely. It is a vague term that needs clarifying and diagnosing.

2. Diagnosis can be difficult because of non-specificity and frequent lack of history from the patient. A third party history is key.

3. Testing—physical and psychological—is necessary to obtain a precise diagnosis and as a foundation for planning and evaluating treatment.

4. There is some value in trying to identify dementia subtypes, reversible causes of cognitive impairment and comorbidities. But the key skills are interpersonal and clinical.

Chapter 3

Delirium

What is delirium?

Delirium is an organic psychiatric syndrome—a psychological or mental response to a 'physical' cause. It comprises a transient, usually reversible state, with variable, fluctuating and wide-ranging abnormalities in attention, alertness, cognition, perception, sleep-wake cycle, agitation or psycho-motor retardation.

The International Classification of Diseases (ICD-10—Box 3.1) requires all of:
- Impairment of consciousness and attention.
- Global disturbance of cognition.
- Psychomotor disturbance.
- Abnormal sleep-wake cycle.
- Emotional disturbance.

The American Psychiatric Association DSM-IV also specifies 'evidence from the history, physical examination, or laboratory findings is present that indicates the disturbance is caused by a direct physiologic conse-quence of a general medical condition, an intoxicating substance, medica-tion use, or more than one cause'.

Box 3.1 WHO ICD-10 criteria for delirium

- Impairment of consciousness and attention, reduced ability to direct, focus, sustain and shift attention.
- Global disturbance of cognition—perceptual distortion, illusions, hallucinations, mostly visual; impaired abstract thinking and compre-hension; immediate recall and recent memory; disorientated in time, sometimes place and person.
- Psychomotor disturbance, hypo or hyperactivity or unpredictable shifting between the two.
- Sleep-wake cycle—insomnia, daytime drowsiness, sleep reversal, symptoms worse at night, disturbing dreams or nightmares which may continue as hallucinations on awakening.
- Emotional disturbance—depression, anxiety, fear, irritability, euphoria, apathy, perplexity.

Prevalence

Prevalence varies with setting, population studied and severity of illness. Prevalence also depends on the severity threshold set for defining delirium.

Arguably all severely physically ill patients are delirious—drowsy, inattentive, forgetful and unable to reason. Published series of intensive care and terminally ill patients give prevalences of 80% and 60% respectively.

Overall in the general hospital 15% of all general medical and surgical inpatients are, or become, delirious. The figure is greater in older patients (perhaps 30% of acute geriatric ward patients), post-operatively (15% overall, 50% post hip fracture surgery), and in patients with prior dementia. Half of those with dementia admitted to general hospitals have superadded delirium, and 25–50% of cases of delirium are on a background of dementia.

Diagnosis

There are two elements:
- The syndrome.
- The cause.

Why is it hard to spot a delirious patient?

Delirium is under-recognized:
- Features vary from patient to patient, and from time to time. Patients may be agitated, hypoactive or depressed. Single assessments are often insufficient.
- It may complicate pre-existing dementia, and distinguishing new deficits from old can be hard. This is especially true in a hospital environment unfamiliar to the patient, which itself leads to disorientation.
- Hypoactive forms are especially difficult to distinguish in delirium complicating dementia.
- It is difficult to distinguish in an ill person (especially on an ITU or in terminal care).
- It can be difficult to describe. Physicians may be reliant on information of uncertain validity (nurse/relative reports).
- Applying cognitive tests is difficult in an agitated or inattentive patient.
- This is generally unfamiliar territory for physicians, relatives and nurses. So they neither anticipate it, nor recognize what they see when it is there.
- Making a diagnosis does not always impact on management (although recognizing delirium may alert you to the seriousness of the problem). The key time to recognize delirium is when it is causing problems (behavioural, engagement with therapy, risk assessing discharge plans), rather than a transient phenomenon that passes when something else is being treated.
- Difficult behaviours induce the wrong frame of mind in staff—who may become angry and confrontational rather than diagnostically curious.
- In settings unfamiliar with delirium, false assumptions are made (often that the patient needs sedating) and multiple or competing causes overlooked (just alcohol or something else as well?).

Features

Delirium is a disorder of:
- Abnormal cognition, 'confusion' (📖 Chapter 2 p. 26–28):
  - Orientation—test person, place, time. Earliest to appear and last to disappear is disorientation to time, especially judgement of the passage of time. But do not expect complete accuracy in someone ill, in an unfamiliar place, possibly moved several times between hospitals or wards, or following a prolonged admission.
  - Memory—registration, retention, and recall may all be abnormal. Test three items after 2 minutes. Afterwards there is usually amnesia for the delirious period.
  - Concentration—inability to focus, sustain, and direct attention. May be evident in conversation. To test, spell 'world', serial sevens, or counting 20–1 backwards. The key feature is distractibility, which may make prolonged cognitive testing impossible.
  - Alternatively you can use the Abbreviated Mental Test or Mini-Mental State Examination (📖 Chapter 13 p. 323), but look to see the pattern of errors as well as the overall score.
  - Testing may be slow as well as inaccurate.
- Impaired consciousness. This means abnormal awareness, alertness, attention, and arousal. Alertness is the ability to respond to external stimuli, and this may be increased (hypervigilant) or decreased (apathetic, disengaged). Impairment varies from barely perceptible mental slowing, uncertainty, or fatigue, to near unconsciousness. There is also inability to select important stimuli and use them in context. Lack of discrimination leads to inattentiveness or distractibility. Failure to shift attention causes perseveration (repetition of verbal or motor activity).

Abnormal cognition and consciousness is:
- Usually fluctuating (mostly over a period of hours; a single clinical assessment will not make the diagnosis, so ask relatives or nurses). At times the patient may appear near normal.
- Acute onset (hours to days, although it is commoner in people with pre-existing dementia). If there is pre-existing dementia, family carers are better than ward staff at identifying the abrupt change in function or mental state.
- Due to an identifiable physical cause (but identifying it can be difficult).
- Reversible with treatment of the physical disease (but this may be slower than you expect—often 2–4 weeks, up to several months).
- Worse at night. At night sleep is short and fragmented, with vivid or frightening dreams. However, remember that in unfamiliar, noisy, disturbed hospital environments sleep is often poor, so many medical patients are tired or sleepy during the day.

Look for:
- Disordered thinking:
  - Incoherence, such as rambling or irrelevant conversation, illogical flow of ideas, poor reasoning, or unpredictable switching from subject to subject. Content of thought varies with time.

- Misperceptions, illusions, and hallucinations. Usually visual and frightening. Typically animated (i.e. formed and moving) e.g. animals or insects. Can also be auditory or tactile. More bizarre experiences may suggest hallucinogenic drugs.
  - Paranoia. Delusions are reported in 50% of delirium cases, but they are often fleeting and not systematized.
- Abnormal appearance and behaviour:
  - May or may not look unwell, agitated, tremulous, or hypoactive.
  - May represent responses to hallucinations or delusions. Activity is purposeless, repetitive or misdirected.
  - Speech may be mumbled or incoherent.
  - In one series of delirious patients, 15% were hyperactive, 19% hypoactive, 52% mixed and 14% neither.
- Mood is labile, perplexed, anxious, or depressed, but thought content has an empty quality. Depression in an elderly medical inpatient is more likely to represent delirium than affective disorder. And physically ill people often have understandably low mood.
- Insight usually lacking.
- Asterixis (a flapping tremor—gently passively dorsiflex the out-stretched wrist and hold it for 10–20 seconds) is seen in metabolic encephalopathies (liver and renal failure) and respiratory failure.
- Often doubly incontinent—this is part of the syndrome, and does not necessarily mean that urinary infection is the cause.

Beware other causes of apparently abnormal cognition:
(p. 18–21, 28)
- Receptive aphasia: test for receptive function first. A complex motor command ('touch your right ear with your left hand') is a reasonable screen. Simple single stage commands ('shut your eyes', 'put out your tongue') may be intact even in severe motor impairment.
- Expressive aphasia: listen to spontaneous speech for hesitancy and word finding difficulties; test naming (increasingly difficult parts of a watch: watch, strap, buckle, hands, winder; or spectacles: spectacles, lens, arm). Mistaking aphasia for 'confusion' is so common that you must routinely consider the possibility.
- Deafness (occasionally 'confusion' or 'receptive aphasia' can be 'cured' by turning on the hearing aid).
- Language—there are many older people in the UK whose first language is not English.
- Bewilderment, belligerence, anger.

Causes

Anyone can become delirious. The best model is to think in terms of pre-disposition and precipitant. In general, the more severe the precipitating factor, and the more acute the onset, the more likely delirium is and the worse its severity will be.

Note that delirium tremens and neuroleptic malignant syndrome may be different (due to chronic neurochemical changes and receptor up-regulation).

Predisposition

- Age—children and the very elderly are most at risk. Possibly due to age-related selective neuronal loss, and a relative cholinergic deficit.
- Chronic brain disease:
  - Dementia is one of the strongest and most consistent risk factors. Underlying dementia is observed in 25–50% of delirious patients. The presence of dementia increases the risk of delirium by 5–10 times.
  - Increased risk is also seen after head injury and stroke.
- Addiction (alcohol, benzodiazepines).
- Visual or hearing impairment.
- Multiple prescribed drugs (which is possibly simply a marker of poor general health) and impaired drug metabolism (e.g. renal failure).
- Psychosocial stress—bereavement, relocation, sleep deprivation, sensory deprivation or overload.

Precipitants

Any medical illness, intoxication, or medication can cause delirium.

However, determining the cause of a delirium is not easy. Delirium may be multifactorial in aetiology—identifying a single potential cause may not be enough. Sometimes (16% of cases) no convincing physical cause is found for a clinically convincing delirium.

Conceptually there are four groups of causes:
1. Brain disorders.
2. Systemic disorders secondarily affecting the brain.
3. Exogenous toxic substances.
4. Withdrawal of drugs.

Brain disorders
- Structural changes:
  - head injury
  - stroke: infarction, intracerebral haemorrhage, subarachnoid haemorrhage, subdural haematoma. Note that TIA is not a cause of confusion.
  - global hypoxia
  - primary or metastatic brain tumour
  - hypertensive encephalopathy
  - cerebral vasculitis.
- Intracranial infection:
  - meningitis
  - encephalitis
  - HSV, other viral, HIV encephalitis
  - brain abscess.

- Epilepsy—post-ictal confusion.
- Toxic encephalopathies (e.g. heavy metals).
- Others, including Wernicke's encephalopathy.

Systemic disorders
- Infections:
  - septicaemia
  - pneumonia
  - urinary tract infections
  - cellulitis
  - intra-abdominal (often masked).
- Metabolic causes:
  - fluid and electrolyte abnormalities (hyponatraemia, hypernatraemia, hypercalcaemia), acid-base disturbances
  - hypoglycaemia, hyperglycaemia
  - hepatic or renal failure
  - severe hypothyroidism, thyroid storm.
- Hypoxic and hypo perfusion states:
  - lung disease
  - shock (septic, cardiogenic, hypovolaemic, pulmonary embolism, drug induced, anaphylactic)
  - left heart failure, cardiac arrhythmias
  - myocardial infarction
  - anaemia (may contribute but unlikely to cause delirium in isolation).
- Hypothermia.

Toxic causes
- Intoxication—alcohol, heroin, cannabis, hallucinogens.
- Drug-induced:
  - antimuscarinic drugs (atropine, tricyclic antidepressants, antipsychotics, antiparkinson drugs, bladder instability drugs, gut antispasmodics, disopyramide)
  - opiates (some seem to be worse than others—codeine and dihydrocodeine in particular)
  - antiparkinson drugs (dopamine agonists e.g. ropinirole; antimuscarinic e.g. trihexyphenidyl; levodopa)
  - sedative hypnotics (benzodiazepines)
  - corticosteroids (especially in very high doses)
  - neuroleptic malignant syndrome.

Substance withdrawal
Typically a few days to a week after cessation—alcohol, opiates, benzodiazepines, selective serotonin re-uptake inhibitors.

Delirium mimics: differential diagnosis

(See Table 3.1)

- Causes of agitation e.g. pain, constipation, lower urinary tract symptoms.
- Dementia with Lewy bodies (also characterized by confusion, fluctuation and hallucinations, almost always with signs of Parkinsonism, but beware extrapyramidal side effects of antipsychotic drugs) (📖 p. 260).
- Progression of vascular dementia (the steps of a 'stepwise decline' include a sudden deterioration).
- Decompensation of pre-existing dementia:
  - disorientation, bewilderment, fear, or agitation in a strange hospital environment
  - a behavioural crisis (due to poor memory or insight, misjudgement, or disinhibition).
- Pure disorders of alertness:
  - drowsiness due to neurological disease (raised intra-cranial pressure, infections, stroke, tumours)
  - sedation due to drugs
  - 'septic encephalopathy'—drowsiness associated with systemic sepsis.
- Disorders of communication (dysphasia, deafness).
- Post-ictal confusion.
- Transient global amnesia (TGA).
- Other primary psychiatric disorders e.g. depression, mania, functional psychosis, schizophrenia (📖 p. 18–21).

Table 3.1 Differentiating delirium from dementia and psychosis

Characteristics	Delirium	Dementia	Acute functional psychosis
Definition	Confusion in a previously well patient, or worsening of chronic confusion, which develops over a short period	Progressive global decline in cognitive function	E.g. schizophrenia, severe depression
Onset	Sudden	Insidious	Sudden
Course over 24 h	Fluctuating, worse at night	Usually stable	Stable
Consciousness	Reduced	Clear	Clear
Attention	Disordered, distractible	Usually normal	May be disordered
Orientation	Usually impaired	Variable	May be impaired
Hallucination	Common	Often absent	Predominantly auditory
Memory	Recent and immediate memory impaired	Recent and remote memory impaired	Variable
Involuntary movements	Often coarse tremor or asterixis	Often absent	Usually absent (except for side effects of drugs)
Physical illness or drug toxicity	Always present	Often absent	Usually absent

Management

- Make the diagnosis.
- Seek, identify and treat the underlying cause (but no cause can be found in 16% of cases of clinically convincing delirium). Retake the history, re-examine the patient (including neurological insofar as this is possible), order laboratory and radiological investigations. Withdraw all suspect drugs.
- Avoid provocation or over-stimulation. Manage in a quiet, well-lit side room. Reasoning, arguing, shouting, admonition, threatening or punishment *never* work.
- Ensure glasses and hearing aids are worn where appropriate.
- Involve relatives in care, and actively support relatives by repeated explanation and reassurance.
- Delirious patients may pull out intravenous lines, climb out of bed, and may not be compliant. Perceptual problems lead to agitation, fear, combative behaviour, and wandering. Avoid using physical restraints. Cot sides (bed rails) do not reduce the incidence of injury, and should be well-padded if used. A hospital bed which lowers to floor level is preferable if the patient is trying to get out of bed.
- Ask for one-to-one nursing ('specialing'; nursing management usually state that this will be provided if required, but may argue whether it is actually required!). This may be cost-effective (if it reduces delirious time and length of stay, and avoids complications, accidents or complaints) and helps minimize the use of chemical and physical restraints.
- Use of sedative drugs:
  - is a last resort
  - to relieve psychosis, agitation or severe distress to the patient
  - to avoid injury or harm to the patient, other patients, staff or relatives
  - to allow medical therapy to be delivered
  - never as a first response
  - never to make up for lack of nursing staff (this is probably illegal)
  - see Table 3.2 for drugs to use in an emergency
  - give drugs time to act (at least 20 minutes per dose increment).
- You must minimize stimulation and provocation at the same time.
- Drugs are legally justified so long as you can argue that your prescription (and other actions without the patient's consent):
  - are the minimum required to control the immediate problem
  - are in the patient's best interests (📖 Chapter 11 Box 11.3 p 288).
- If you decide a regular sedative drug is required, use one with which you are familiar. For example haloperidol (start with 500 mcg bd to tds, increasing to 2 mg or 5 mg tds); risperidone (500 mcg–1 mg bd); sulpiride (100 mg at night or bd, increasing to 200 mg bd); lorazepam (500 mcg od or bd, increasing to 1mg bd or (rarely) 2 mg bd). Review daily.
- If first line measures fail, seek more senior advice.
- Nursing confused patients is difficult and wearing. Be sympathetic and supportive.

- Junior doctors should take nurses' advice on what the problem might be and what might help, without being pushed into over-prescription of sedative drugs. But don't accept vague descriptions (e.g. 'confused'), press them to be specific (e.g. resisting nursing care).

Box 3.2 Management of delirium

- Find the cause.
- Treat it. Stop potential culprit drugs.
- Keep your nerve.
- Assess disability—mobility, falls, continence, behaviour.
- Treat comorbidity.
- Antipsychotics only to prevent physical harm:
  - manage without if at all possible; usually it is
  - avoid provocation and over-stimulation
  - reasoning, threats, and punishment never work.
- Minimize neuroleptic and antidepressant use.
- Explain delirium to relatives and patients when they recover.
- Don't make the wrong plans too soon.

Caution

- Elderly patients may be exquisitely sensitive to sedative drugs.
- Always start with small doses and titrate as necessary.
- Avoid antipsychotic drugs in patients with DLB.
- Haloperidol has a half-life of up to 60 h in older people. Drug clearance time (5 × half-life) can therefore be up to a week.

Table 3.2 Drugs for emergency control of severely disturbed behaviour

Patient group	Try first	Try second	Maximum dose in first 6 h
Already on depot/regular high-dose antipsychotics	Lorazepam 2 mg IM	Repeat lorazepam, then try haloperidol 5 mg IM	Lorazepam 4 mg + haloperidol 18 mg
Acute alcoholic withdrawal	Lorazepam 2 mg IM	Repeat	Lorazepam 8 mg
Frail elderly or severe respiratory disease	Haloperidol 2.5 mg IM	Lorazepam 1 mg IM	Lorazepam 4 mg + haloperidol 10 mg
Highly aroused, physically robust, adult	Lorazepam 2 mg IM + haloperidol 5 mg IM	Repeat	Lorazepam 4 mg + haloperidol 18 mg

These doses are in excess of the SPC; however, NICE acknowledges that there may be certain circumstances where this is appropriate.

When should you seek psychiatric assistance?

Managing delirium should be within the expert repertoire of geriatricians, but all physicians will come across delirium and their levels of expertise will vary. The interests of patients are best served by their being managed, or given opinions, by those with appropriate expertise. Those without expertise should ask for help when they know they have reached their limits, but should be expected to offer some assessment and effort in determining the diagnosis. Not every case of delirium is caused by urinary tract infection.

If a confident diagnosis of delirium has been made, it may be as appropriate for the general physician to ask for a geriatrician's opinion as a psychiatrist's.

A psychiatrist (or psychiatric liaison nurse) can help:
• If the diagnosis is uncertain, or may be complicated by comorbid psychiatric illness.
• Advise on treatment, especially of severe behavioural disturbance.
• Advise and assess for compulsory detention under mental health legislation. This will rarely be appropriate in delirium (although in England & Wales this may change with the Deprivation of Liberty amendments to the Mental Capacity Act).
• Support general ward staff (doctors and nurses) and relatives— coaching on behavioural approaches, assurance that the correct management is being pursued.

Investigations

Table 3.3 Investigations

What?	Why?	Comments
Full blood count	Infection, severe anaemia	Also gives clues to other systemic disease e.g. renal failure, malignancy.
ESR	Infection, inflammatory, malignant conditions	Can be moderately raised in well elderly people. Often leads to multiple follow-up tests.
CRP	Infection, inflammatory, malignant conditions	More sensitive, specific and sensitive to change than ESR.
U&E (Na, K, urea, creatinine)	Electrolyte disturbance, renal failure	Hypo or hypernatraemia
Glucose	Hypoglycaemia, hyperglycaemia	Hypoglycaemia seen with insulin or sulphonylurea therapy (insulinoma is rare).
Calcium	Hypercalcaemia	Main causes: hyperparathyroidism, malignancy, myeloma
Liver function	Hepatic encephalopathy, clue to systemic disease	
B12, folate	Associated with cognitive impairment	Unlikely to present as delirium
Thyroid function	'Myxoedema madness', thyrotoxicosis	Abnormalities common, note 'sick euthyroid'—test abnormalities in systemic disease not due to thyroid dysfunction.
Blood alcohol	Acute intoxication	
Drug assays	Toxic level, compliance	Including illicit, if appropriate, blood and urine.
CXR	Infection, heart failure, malignancy	Often technically inadequate in ill or agitated patients.
Urine dipstick (nitrites, leucocyte esterase), culture	Infection	
Blood culture	Infection	Including endocarditis
CT head/MRI	Tumour, subdural, cerebrovascular disease	Certainly if trauma or focal neurological signs, also when no other good explanation has been found.
CSF	Meningitis, encephalitis, malignancy	

CT, US abdomen	Abscess, malignancy	
CT thorax	Infection, malignancy, fibrosis, pulmonary embolism	
EEG	Seizures, CJD	Non-specifically abnormal in delirium. Useful to exclude sub-clinical status epilepticus. Abnormal EEG with normal structural imaging highly suggestive of DLB.
Pulse oximetry	Hypoxia	
ECG	Arrhythmias, ischaemia	

Special situations

Delirium tremens (DTs)

This is a severe withdrawal reaction after cessation of habitual heavy alcohol intake, with physical and psychiatric features. It occurs 3–10 days after the last drink. Only 5% of chronic heavy drinkers develop DTs on cessation.

In the full syndrome:

- Florid hallucinations and illusions, visual and auditory (typically animated visual forms, such as insects, birds or rats) and formication (tactile hallucinations, usually of crawling insects), delusions.
- Impairment of consciousness.
- Autonomic over-activity (tremor, hypertension, tachycardia, sweating, vomiting, fever).
- Agitation, anxiety, or terror.
- Withdrawal seizures occur within 6–48 h of alcohol cessation. In 60% of patients the seizures are multiple, and 3% develop status epilepticus. 30–40% of patients with alcohol withdrawal seizures progress to DTs.
- Mortality is 5–15% (respiratory failure, arrhythmias and seizures).
- There is no alcohol craving in the acute episode.

Less severe versions with confusion, tremor and hallucinations are more common.

Minor withdrawal occurs within 6–24 h following the last drink and is characterized by tremor, anxiety, nausea, vomiting, and insomnia. Half of chronic heavy alcohol users will experience withdrawal symptoms on cessation.

Beware superadded infection (half have pneumonia), head injury, hypoglycaemia, liver failure, Wernicke's encephalopathy, refeeding syndrome, and recreational drug use.

In established DTs, management requires control with intravenous long-acting benzodiazepines (diazepam or chlordiazepoxide), often in large doses. Prevention entails oral benzodiazepines (e.g. chlordiazepoxide 20 mg qds, tailing down over a week). High-dose parenteral B vitamins should also be given to avert the risk of Wernicke's encephalopathy.

Neuroleptic malignant syndrome

This is an uncommon cause of delirium but important to recognize. It is caused by antipsychotic (dopamine antagonist) drugs, and therefore usually occurs as an apparent intercurrent physical illness in a psychiatric patient. It usually occurs after starting the drug or increasing the dose, and on higher doses. There is agitation, hyperpyrexia, increased muscle tone, autonomic instability (tachycardia, sweating, labile blood pressure, urinary incontinence) and greatly increased serum creatine kinase (CK).

Management comprises withdrawal of the culprit drug, cardiovascular supportive (intravenous fluids), excluding or treating comorbidity (infection), consideration of some specific therapies in difficult cases (intravenous dantrolene), and reconsideration of how to manage the psychiatric problem that prompted the use of neuroleptics in the first place. Resolution occurs over 1–2 weeks.

On making (or even considering) the diagnosis, potential culprit drugs should be immediately withdrawn. In practice this is often more difficult than it sounds. A psychiatrically ill (often elderly) person becomes more physically unwell with a fever and tachycardia. The first thought is to diagnose infection (common) rather than NMS (rare). Thinking about the diagnosis and ordering a serum CK is the key. The patient will usually need intravenous hydration, and possibly a urinary catheter.

Behaviour (agitation) may become more difficult with NMS, or re-emerge as a problem as the NMS resolves in the absence of sedative drugs. The situation will often be further complicated by a discussion about where the patient should be managed. Too physically ill for a psychiatric ward, too psychiatrically ill for a medical ward, with a condition with which most physicians will be unfamiliar. A good acute geriatric medical or neurology ward should be able to cope.

If neuroleptic medication is still required there is a problem. Neuroleptics 'cross react'—there are likely to be problems with all if there have been problems with one. Re-introduce the drug at ultra-low doses, and keep a close watch for pyrexia and increased CK. Alternatively try something different, such as a benzodiazepine or the sedating antidepressant mirtazapine, depending on the indication.

Wernicke's encephalopathy

This is a syndrome of delirium, eye movement disorder, ataxia, nystagmus, and Korsakoff's psychosis. Korsakoff's psychosis is a syndrome of antegrade and retrograde amnesia with confabulation (plausible fabricated information filling in gaps in memory). These spell out the mnemonic DRANK if you make the eye movement disorder into 'rectus palsy'. It is caused by thiamine deficiency, usually in association with chronic sub-nutrition in alcoholism. But it is also seen after refeeding, especially with carbohydrates, after prolonged starvation in other settings (swallowing disorder, bowel disorders). Eye movement problems are often said to be pathognomonic, but in a series of pathologically-defined cases, mostly undiagnosed in life, non-specific 'confusion' was the commonest feature.

Have a low threshold for giving oral thiamine (100 mg tds for a week) to confused patients. In alcoholism gut absorption may be poor, so in these patients, or if clinical suspicion of the syndrome is high, give parenteral B vitamins. Other nutritional deficiencies (e.g. magnesium, phosphate, and folate) may complicate the picture further ('refeeding syndrome'—rhabdomyolysis, heart and respiratory failure, arrhythmias or seizures).

HIV encephalopathy and HIV associated dementia (HAD)

Neuropsychiatric problems will be the presenting feature of HIV infection in 10–20% of cases. Delirium, often with additional motor abnormalities, may occur acutely at HIV seroconversion (HIV encephalopathy).

Chronic and progressive HAD also occurs, along with a more common but minimally disabling variant, minor cognitive motor disorder (MCMD), which will ultimately progress to dementia (☐ Chapter 15 p. 360). In these conditions cognitive impairment is associated with language disturbance, apraxia, and various motor abnormalities including weakness, tremor, and clumsiness.

Cognitive problems in HIV disease, especially those of sudden onset or that are rapidly progressive, may also be due to opportunistic infections, tumours, or drugs. These include lymphoma, Kaposi's sarcoma, progressive multifocal leucoencephalopathy, cryptococcal and tuberculous meningitis, and drug side effects. Urgent imaging and other investigation is required.

Post-operative confusion

Numerous features contribute to post-operative delirium:

- Emergency surgery is done on ill people—often with associated intra-abdominal sepsis, or major trauma (hip fractures). As well as sepsis, there may be hypotension, anaemia, fluid deprivation or overload, electrolyte disturbance, or loss of diabetic control. Anaesthetic and analgesic drugs, especially opiates, are potent causes of delirium.

- Complications including chest and urinary infections (sometimes associated with urinary catheterization), pulmonary embolism, and pressure sores may contribute. Moreover, an acute physical illness (such as pneumonia, heart attack, or stroke) may have precipitated a fall that caused a fracture, or an advanced cancer may have caused a bowel obstruction. Prior comorbidities complicate further. Heart failure and chronic lung disease risk hypoxia. Chronic renal failure and nephrotoxic drugs (non-steroidal anti-inflammatories, ACE inhibitors, gentamicin) along with hypotension and fluid balance problems risk acute renal failure.

- Unfortunately, surgical wards are organized for delivering interventions on generally-well people and confusion can be met with neither sympathy nor expertise in its investigation and management. But there is nothing fundamentally different about post-operative delirium.

- Beware undiagnosed dementia becoming evident about the time of elective or emergency surgery. The social facade may be sufficient to cause the busy surgeon to fail to recognize well-compensated cognitive impairment on initial assessment of an elective problem, or even whilst gaining consent, especially if many of the practical details are arranged by supportive family members. However, disruption of the usual environment and routine can be cruelly revealing of loss of cognitive and adaptive powers.

- So evaluation of a confused surgical patient requires immediate assessment, observation over time, and the taking of a proper third party cognitive history. The third party history should be taken immediately—and may conveniently be added in to a discussion with family about what is happening with the patient.

- Look first at drugs (opiates, antimuscarinic) and for infection (wound, chest, urine, abscess) or hypoxia. Next look for a metabolic cause (electrolytes, renal function, glucose, calcium). Then consider perioperative heart attack, rhythm disturbance, stroke, or PE. Consider whether pain, urinary retention, or constipation might be contributing.

Prevention

- Most prevention is good, common sense nursing and medicine for older people. Do all the usual, simple things thoroughly and well.
- Identify at risk patients and treat early and aggressively for their medical illnesses. Preventative measures appear to be as effective in people with prior dementia as in those without.
- Know your risk situations (post-operative, terminal care, people with dementia in hospital) and increase vigilance.
- Avoid culprit drugs and polypharmacy. Of all the things we do in medicine, stopping and starting drugs is the easiest to change. Make sure every drug is justified.
  - is there a clear indication? (e.g. diuretics, proton pump inhibitors)
  - is the drug one that is known to have a limited duration of effectiveness? (e.g. benzodiazepine and related hypnotics)
  - has response to the drug been assessed and determined to be beneficial? (e.g. antidepressants, analgesics)
  - is there reasonable evidence that the patient (and his or her supporter and helpers) can take all the drugs reliably? If not, compromise, stop any 'optional extras' (e.g. preventative drugs with high numbers needed to treat)
  - in at-risk patients avoid completely, if possible, antimuscarinic, dopamine agonists, and the worst of the opiates (dihydrocodeine, codeine)
- Consider structured programmes of delirium avoidance (see Box 3.3).

Box 3.3 Prevention of delirium

- 853 general medical inpatients aged over 70 participated in a trial. One intervention, two control units, enrollment by prospective matching.
- Standardized protocols for managing six risk factors for delirium:
  - Cognition: orientation protocol (board with staff names and daily schedule, enhanced communication) three times a day if MMSE <20, once a day otherwise. Therapeutic activities protocol (current events, reminiscence, word games) three times a day.
  - Sleep: noise reduction strategy, non-pharmacological intervention (drink, music, massage).
  - Immobility: ambulation or active range of motion exercises three times a day. Avoidance of urinary catheters and restraints.
  - Vision: if VA <20/70 (6/20), visual aids and adaptive equipment provided (large-print books, telephone keypad, fluorescent bell pull), daily instruction on use.
  - Hearing: if <6/12 whispers heard, use portable amplifier, earwax disimpaction, special communication, daily instruction on use.
  - Dehydration: if urea/creatinine ratio >70 (SI units), dehydration protocol (mainly pushing oral fluids).
- Delirium was assessed daily. It developed in 10% of the intervention group and 15% of controls (OR 0.60, 95% CI 0.39–0.92). 62 vs 90 delirious episodes; 105 d vs 161 d. Intervention was also associated with improved cognition amongst those impaired at admission, but did not affect delirium severity or recurrence.
- The interventions were simple and thoroughly applied, but very labour intensive.

Inouye, S. et al., *NEJM* 1999; **340**: 669–76

Course and prognosis

There is limited evidence. The question of prognosis is hard to define because it is so dependent on how delirium is diagnosed, and the severity of both the delirium and the underlying physical illness.

Mild and transient cases incidental to an appropriately managed physical illness are usually not specifically diagnosed, and have commensurately good outcomes. Delirium in an intensive care unit or in terminal care has a grave outlook driven by the physical illness. Outcome in delirium complicating dementia is worse than that in delirium alone.

On treating the physical illness delirium recovers, but recovery may be slower than anticipated and making erroneous (relatively) hasty decisions is a major risk (about future hospital discharge and care arrangements e.g. care home placement). Recovery takes days to weeks, and most (but not all) recover within a month. Recovery time is more prolonged in more severe cases. By arbitrary definition, if the disturbance has not recovered within 6 months, it doesn't count as delirium.

In a systematic review of psychiatrically-diagnosed cases (including 8 studies and 573 patients):
- After 1 month, 14% had died, 47% were institutionalized, and 55% improved mentally.
- Compared with unmatched controls, length of hospital stay was longer, mortality was higher, and more were institutionalized, at 1 and 6 months.
- Poorer outcomes were associated with dementia and severe physical illness.
  Selection bias is highly likely to have distorted these figures.
  In acute general hospital practice, as a ballpark figure, 15–30% die.

Amongst survivors both physical and mental disability is common.

Failure of delirium to recover

A particularly difficult situation is 'delirium' that appears not to recover. Reassess the situation: is the diagnosis of delirium correct? Have all appropriate and reasonable tests for a cause been done? There are three main possibilities here:
- Previously undiagnosed dementia presenting in crisis (intercurrent illness or decompensation). Usually hints about prior memory lapses or avoidance of mentally challenging tasks will be elicited in the cognitive history. However, sometimes these will be denied or explained away as 'normal for age' and compensated for by spouse or other relatives.
- Previously undiagnosed dementia presenting with delirium, and only partial recovery of cognition.
- Progression of vascular dementia. In its most extreme form this is seen in persisting cognitive impairment after acute stroke in someone with no prior cognitive impairment—as occurs in perhaps 20% of first strokes. Other acute neurological emergencies (such as head injury, vasculitis, brain tumour or hypoxia) may have persisting deficits in the same way. In someone carrying a burden of 'silent' cerebrovascular disease, a new infarct may appear as an acute decline in cognition that fails to recover fully.

Long-term prognosis

A related issue is long-term prognosis, in particular the long-term risk of dementia. Those suffering an episode of delirium are three times more likely to become demented than controls. This makes sense if we propose an aetiological model in which delirium results from a pathophysiological disturbance that overwhelms 'cerebral reserve' or perhaps 'cholinergic reserve'. Those developing delirium are likely to have compromised 'reserve'. Superimposing progressive neuro-degeneration or cerebrovascular disease over time will further compromise cognitive function, to the point where the 'dementia threshold' is reached.

Summary

1. Delirium is a disorder of cognition, consciousness, and attention due to a physical cause.
2. Delirium is one of the 'geriatric giants'—non-specific presentations of any acute illness. It may be precipitated by any neurological, medical or drug cause, or by withdrawal of some drug classes.
3. Some people (e.g. those with dementia) and situations (e.g. post-operative) pose especially high risk of delirium.
4. Delirium may be over-active or hypoactive, is variable, and is worse at night. Diagnosis needs prolonged observation or reports of the same. Hallucinations, delusions, misperceptions, fear, and depression are common.
5. Investigate thoroughly. There may be multiple causes and aggravating factors.
6. Management involves treating the underlying cause, whilst providing supportive care and avoiding complications and accidents. Avoid sedative drugs unless required for severe distress or danger to the patient or others.
7. Good nursing and medical care can reduce the incidence of delirium.
8. Prognosis is mixed. Delirium is often precipitated by severe illness, or occurs when there is severe underlying illness (like advanced cancer), which carries its own poor prognosis for survival. Otherwise recovery usually occurs in days to weeks (but can take up to 3 months or more). People who suffer delirium are more likely to develop subsequent dementia.

Chapter 4

Care

'Care' and 'treatment' in dementia

To care is to be concerned or responsible for someone, to protect them or do things for them. The use of the terms 'care' and 'treatment' in relation to dementia requires some explanation.

In some fields, the term 'care' implies a somewhat passive form of activity—merely a 'looking after', perhaps to allow the serious work of 'treatment' to impact on prognosis and well-being. With dementia these roles are reversed, with quality of care being the most significant single determinant of both cognitive and non-cognitive outcomes. In this context, we might say that care *is* the most important aspect of treatment of dementia.

In the early stages of dementia, care will usually be provided by family members and friends. Later, professional staff are more likely to become involved. The principles outlined here apply to everyone who cares for people with dementia.

Supporting carers

Spending hours at a time with someone who is confused, and who can easily become anxious, distressed, angry, or determined, has a significant impact on the well-being of carers. Their capacity to remain empathic and supportive will be partly determined by their own personality and the nature of their relationship with the person with dementia, but will always be diminished if they do not receive sufficient support and understanding (as well as breaks) themselves.

For professional carers, the prospect of seeing their work rewarded by 'recovery' is denied. Skill, kindness, and compassion can be quickly forgotten and often misinterpreted.

For family carers there can be the difficult task of mourning lost aspects of a relationship in the midst of striving to maintain whatever quality of life is still possible.

For both there is an awareness of the low esteem and status associated with personal care and the drudgery of repetitive task routines. Caring for those who are becoming increasingly dependent can evoke strong negative feelings towards the person who is being cared for, and these can in turn lead to feelings of shame and guilt. In the absence of sufficient support for carers, these tendencies will often lead to their erecting rigid defences that diminish their capacity to remain in emotional contact with the person with dementia.

Promoting independence—avoiding failure

A key aspect of the art of dementia care is achieving a balance between promoting independence and minimizing experience of failure. As cognitive impairment attacks a person's abilities and skill levels across a range of activities, it is all too tempting for carers to accelerate this decline by 'taking over' and doing things themselves. Lack of confidence may lead the person with dementia to collude with this 'disempowerment' so that a vicious cycle of apathy and inactivity are set in train. This can happen insidiously even in the absence of intent.

A close working knowledge of the areas of retained ability and the degree of assistance required for successful task completion is invaluable.

Carers need to be mindful of fluctuations in levels of functioning, which require constant reassessment.

Flexibility is also helpful—something that is at a premium in more rigid institutional regimes—as Mr. A's willingness to have a shave may not appear until 3:30 p.m. and then again just after 8 p.m., having remained stubbornly absent during the morning period when he would usually have shaved in the past.

Activities of daily living

Principles underpinning good practice

Developmental significance

Good practice in supporting people with activities of daily living (ADLs) is underpinned by an awareness of the potential emotional significance of an increasing dependence on others. ADLs generally involve abilities that are gained in early childhood and are so intrinsic to the status of being an independent, autonomous adult that they are scarcely recognized as skills. The loss of the ability to independently dress, use the toilet, or feed oneself has a devastating impact on a person's self-esteem and image of themselves as an adult. The response of carers will be a key factor in determining the extent of that devastation.

Process, not product

During our working lives the completion of ADLs is often reduced to the level of a necessary task related to a particular goal, enabling us to focus attention on the various projects and activities that occupy our work or leisure time. Thus bathing becomes a means to cleanliness, and eating a route to adequate nutrition.

Good quality dementia care is as concerned with the quality of the experience of carrying out an ADL as it is with its successful completion. Eating and drinking, or bathing, can be opportunities for sensory and social enjoyment. Choosing the clothes one is to wear for the day can be an occasion for asserting one's identity, reminiscing, or expressing a mood.

Having sufficient time is essential to adopting an unhurried approach and the extent of other demands on carer's time will obviously affect this. Institutional life, however, has a tendency to impose its own pace and rhythm in a way that adds unnecessarily to time pressures. The entire complex of systems and routines in a caring environment may need to be reviewed to ensure that the institution is serving the needs of the people in its care, rather than the other way around.

Know the individual, encourage choice

Carers are in a better position to gain an accurate picture of functional abilities than professionals who have briefer, often somewhat artificial, opportunities for observation and testing. A number of scales are available—such as the Bristol ADL (📖 Chapter 13 p 331)—which can be a useful way of summarizing the collective observations of paid and family carers.

The degree of assistance required with different tasks will vary. As a general rule it is helpful to establish the degree of intervention necessary for each activity. Wherever possible the emphasis should be on doing with, in preference to doing for. Assistance should be pitched at a level that compensates for any deficits (sensory and physical as well as cognitive) whilst allowing opportunity to exercise surviving skills and abilities.

Most of us have long-established habits in our ADLs. We tend, for example, to put our clothes on in a certain order, or have particular 'rituals' and preferences in the bathroom. Someone with dementia becomes increasingly reliant upon such routines as they struggle to adapt to new circumstances, and it helps if carers are aware of them.

Equally important is an awareness of an individual's tastes and preferences. A person may be able make a choice of the deodorant/perfume/aftershave they use, or may be reliant on others to know their well-established preferences.

Personal hygiene

- Assess the level of risk for each activity e.g. check the person is able to judge how to run a bowl of water at a safe temperature.
- Establish whether verbal prompts only—such as reminding which step comes next—are required.
- Are some physical prompts needed—such as handing the person a towel when it's time for them to dry themselves?
- If fuller assistance is needed, seek as much co-operation as the person is able to give—e.g. ask if he can lift up his chin in order to allow you to shave his neck.
- Remember that washing, shaving, and dental care are all things that most of us have managed independently and in privacy for many years.
- People with dementia may experience increases in sensation and become very sensitive; their resistance may reflect that they are suffering some physical pain.
- It is helpful to have in mind the degree of support a person will need and to prepare the environment in advance:
  - is the room warm enough?
  - is everything that will be required (shaving gear, toothbrush, towels etc.) to hand?
- Embarrassment and humiliation will be minimized if the carer is calm, prepared, and able to take the required time.

Dressing

- If supervision only is required, make sure clothes are as clean as necessary. Join in with checking over appearance before going to breakfast.
- Is verbal prompting needed, such as discussing preferred choice of clothes, or reminding which item is to be put on next?
- Physical prompts may include laying out the items in order or handing the person the clothes that are to be put on next. It may mean assisting with buttons etc. that are beyond the person's fine motor skills.
- If the person is able to put on single items but struggles with sequencing the overall task of dressing, put out their clothes for them in a pile with the first items to be put on at the top and so on.
- Consider replacing articles if they require complicated fine motor co-ordination, such as shoe laces (elastic laces may help), belts, small buttons etc.

- If full assistance is necessary, ask if they can lift up their foot in order for you to put their sock on.
- Choice of clothing may need to be restricted to either/or when the demand to choose between multiple options becomes overwhelming.
- Diminishing capacity to distinguish between clean and dirty clothes may require the surreptitious (during sleep or at bath-time) removal of favoured but dirty clothes for laundry. A constant demand to wear the same clothes may be met by buying more than one version of the same outfit.
- Be mindful again of the need for privacy and dignity.

Eating and drinking

The middle stages of dementia present a number of challenges to the need to maintain a healthy and balanced diet. These range from difficulties in remembering how much food or fluid has previously been taken to an impaired ability to manage cutlery.

Other problems—such as swallowing difficulties (dysphagia), loss of appetite, and the total loss of ability to put food or drink to one's mouth—tend to appear at a later stage (📖 Chapter 10 p 268) but can occur earlier in some individuals, especially those with a vascular dementia. A referral should be made to a speech and language therapist if dysphagia is compromising nutritional intake.

In general, it is safe to assume that some form of monitoring of intake will be required at some stage. Monitoring weight is a minimum requirement and the use of food and fluid intake charts is justified if there is particular concern or if there is a need to compare the efficacy of different approaches (e.g. snacking/finger foods versus regular larger meals).

Weight loss is a very common problem in all forms of dementia and losses of more than 5% in one month, or 10% in 6 months, should trigger further investigations or prompt referral to a dietician. Dietary supplements are available in a variety of forms to boost nutritional intake.

Dehydration can arise undetected if carers are not vigilant of the need to promote adequate fluid intake. Carers should be alert to indicators of dehydration—headache, increased confusion, lethargy, decreased skin elasticity, hypotension, and tachycardia. Decreased urinary output is expected, but increased urinary frequency may paradoxically occur, as concentrated urine irritates the bladder.

The emphasis is on maximizing enjoyment of eating, the potential for participation, promoting the use of remaining skills, and enabling independence. Food and fluid intake tend to improve when people eat with others in a familiar mealtime setting—i.e. seated at dining tables with a small number of others (although some may find the presence of others too distracting). Appetite is diminished when there is a sense of pressure or being rushed, and distractions such as extraneous noise and activity should be kept to a minimum. Seating and posture need attention as physical discomfort or anxiety will inhibit intake.

When necessary, carers should be prepared to experiment and adapt their approach to nutrition by being flexible about the times of day that people eat, what they eat, and how they eat it. It is worth considering 'cues' that stimulate appetite and a preparedness to eat—such as the smell of cooking food and assisting with the setting of tables.

Increasingly carers will be required to provide supervision, encouragement, and practical help in ensuring adequate food and fluid intake.

Dyspraxia (📖 Chapter 1 p 4–5)

Dyspraxia impairs an individual's ability to manage the practical tasks involved in eating and drinking—such as successful manipulation of cutlery and drinking vessels. Embarrassment at these difficulties and the consequent mess created often leads to reduced opportunities for social eating and drinking, which can impact on social status and self-esteem. Advice from an occupational therapist can identify specific measures.

What can help?
- Finger foods.
- Adapted cutlery that is easier to manipulate.
- Plates with rims, or shallow pasta bowls.
- Non-slip place mats.
- Clear visual contrast between plate/bowl and mat/tablecloth (preferably plain).
- Minimizing unnecessary distracting items on the table.
- Adapted cups/mugs with extra handles and/or a spout.
- Wearing an apron to protect clothing.

If someone needs to be fed
- Ensure good sitting posture and comfort.
- Sit at, or slightly below, eye level and either in front of or slightly at the side of the individual.
- Maintain eye contact.
- Talk to the individual about what is on their plate e.g. 'the cottage pie looks nice'.
- Give small mouthfuls—about a teaspoonful—but enough that they can feel the food in their mouth.
- Discourage talking with food in the mouth due to risk of choking.
- Present food from below the chin, so they have to move their head slightly down to take the food.
- Keep the spoon flat—don't tip it as you withdraw as this will encourage the individual's head to tip up.
- If chewing is difficult, mash or evenly blend food.
- Repeated coughing, choking, or gurgling when taking fluids may mean the fluid needs to be thickened.

Agitation

It can be very difficult for some people with dementia to remain seated for a sustained period of time in order to complete a meal. Appetite decreases when people are agitated and those who are mobile can burn off a significant number of calories over a 24 h period, increasing the potential for weight loss.

What can help?
- Some people prefer to eat alone when agitated.
- Carers should aim for 'little and often' rather than adopting a meal-centred approach to nutrition.

- Leaving 'finger foods', which are known to appeal, in strategic places that the person is likely to come across whilst moving about.
- The use of background music that the person with dementia finds soothing. Music is personal and the carer's tastes may not match those of the person with dementia.

Concentration

As impairment progresses some people lose the ability to concentrate on the task of eating.

What can help?

- Eating with others provides cues and prompts that enhance the potential to persevere with the activity of eating.
- Allowing longer periods of time to complete meals, serving (repeated) smaller portions so that they do not go too cold, and warming crockery before use.

Changes in taste and appetite

Age-related reductions in the senses of taste and smell can be exaggerated in dementia and impair appetite, as can factors such as depression, constipation, and under-activity. Less commonly, some people experience increases in appetite, most often a heightened desire for sweet or salty foods. The subtleties of taste are lost, textures become increasingly important, and people with dementia may lose their appetite for meat.

What can help?

- Maximizing the presence of appetite stimulants such as visual presentation and smell.
- Adding flavour enhancers (but avoid excessive use of salt).
- Providing preferred foods, but be aware that these may change.
- Increased exercise and fresh air.
- Being involved in the preparation of meals.
- Care with textures—avoid lumpy foods or those that require a lot of chewing.

Other reversible contributors to dietary problems

Problems with dentures, tooth decay, and abscesses can all increase the resistance to eating, as can oral thrush.

Some medications, including cholinesterase inhibitors and antidepressants, can cause nausea and loss of appetite. Antimuscarinic drugs cause dry mouth.

'Medical' causes of weight loss

Carers also need to be aware of medical causes of weight loss, including:

- Cancer.
- Thyrotoxicosis.
- Hypercalcaemia.
- Dysphagia (mechanical or neurogenic).

- Malabsorption.
- Infections, especially TB.
- Constipation.
- Diarrhoeal diseases (inflammatory bowel disease).
- Any cause of severe breathlessness ('cardiac cachexia').
- Peptic ulceration (especially with pyloric obstruction).
- Opiate drugs (inhibit appetite).

Toileting (📖 Chapter 9)

Problems with elimination most commonly begin to appear in the middle stages of dementia. One or more of the primary symptoms of dementia may be implicated, making a detailed assessment both necessary and complex—as the measures required to improve the situation are determined by the nature of the contributing factors.

As with other aspects of daily living, carers have to strike a balance between the need to promote independence and maintain skills, and the need to minimize mess, smell, experiences of failure, shame, and humiliation. Awareness (and if possible establishment) of regular patterns of elimination ('prompted voiding', every 2 or 3 h) and of individual behavioural indicators of a need to use the toilet are invaluable aids to making difficulties more manageable.

As the dementia becomes more advanced, the emphasis will shift towards keeping the person as clean and dry as possible through intervention by carers and utilizing incontinence pads and other aids.

'Medical' approaches to managing incontinence (e.g. drugs or operations) are relatively unsuccessful; prompting and behavioural strategies are more important. Remember that unless the bladder is not emptying, urinary catheterization for incontinence should be a last resort, only undertaken after full assessment and consultation.

Non-cognitive contributors

Continence may be affected by features that are not associated with dementia. Is there:
- Urinary tract infection (UTI)?
- Constipation with overflow?
- Medication contributing to the difficulties? (📖 Chapter 9 Table 9.1)

Disorientation

Inability to locate the toilet, particularly in unfamiliar surroundings or at night, often combines with ineffective 'help-seeking' to bring about the initial occurrence of urinary incontinence.

What can help?

- Toilets that are clearly identified (pictures on doors are preferable to words).
- Toilet doors being left ajar so that the toilet, and its availability, can be seen from outside.
- Leaving lights on in toilets at night.
- Commodes, especially near the bed at night-time.

- Awareness of the behavioural indicators of a need to eliminate.
- Offering assistance and enquiring about need for the toilet if the person appears to be searching.
- Prompted voiding.

Agnosia

An inability to recognize appropriate receptacles can lead men in particular to urinate in unacceptable places.

What can help?

- Observation of behavioural indicators as above.
- Removal of potential receptacles that are repeatedly used—although if the likely consequence is urinating on the carpet, it may be preferable to focus on a reasonably hygienic use of the inappropriate receptacle.

Dyspraxia

This presents a challenge to the ability to organize and carry out a number of the skilled tasks involved in toileting, including adjusting clothing and attending to personal hygiene.

What can help?

- Toilet doors that are easy to open and toilet roll dispensers that are familiar.
- Replacement of aspects of clothing—most commonly buttons, zips, and braces—by Velcro fasteners; trousers and skirts with elastic waistbands.
- Encouraging men to urinate when sitting on the toilet, as opposed to standing.
- Practical physical assistance with:
  - adjusting clothing
  - bottom wiping after opening bowels
  - washing hands on completion.
- Advanced planning if practical assistance is required outside the usual care environment. Carers will need to plan access to appropriate toilet facilities (in terms of sufficient space and access for different genders) and any equipment required.
- The RADAR key: this permits access to more than 7000 public toilets with facilities for people with disabilities in the UK. (http://www.radar.org.uk/)

Dysphasia

Communication difficulties complicate an individual's willingness or ability to seek assistance with toileting.

What can help?

- Anticipating when toilet use is likely.
- Observing for signs of agitation or discomfort.
- Asking about need to use the toilet in clear, uncomplicated language in a discreet setting.

Neurogenic detrusor over-activity

Involuntary contractions of the bladder muscle can lead to urinary incontinence (usually in the later stages of dementia), which may not be accompanied by a sense of urgency. In the presence of dysphasia, this can be difficult to differentiate from the loss of the ability to translate a sense of urgency into a purposeful attempt at toileting.

Incontinence aids
Pads and pants

Absorbent pads with specially designed fixation pants to minimize leakage can be worn. Specialist assessment will determine the quantity and size of pads required, which may vary between day and night-time use. These are most suitable for women, who are often unaware of the leakage of small volumes of urine. In men, determined efforts to pass urine in a normal manner may be frustrated by extra layers complicating undressing, or basic anatomy causing the urine stream to miss the pad.

Protective coverings

These can be obtained for mattresses, duvets, pillows, and chairs, and are widely available from department stores and pharmacies. They usually consist of an absorbent side and a waterproof side so as to maximize protection without posing a threat to the person's skin.

Psychological consequences of incontinence

Professional carers should be aware of the feelings of shame and humiliation that accompany the experience of incontinence. Mastering toileting skills is a crucial developmental task in infancy and their loss represents a powerful challenge to anybody's self-esteem.

For family carers, becoming actively involved in the management of a partner's or a parent's toileting needs can profoundly alter the dynamics of their relationship.

Communication

For a person with dementia, the progressive dysphasia that accompanies most types of the disorder can make it feel as if their mother tongue is gradually becoming like a foreign language (□ Box 4.1). This can obviously have an isolating effect. Communicating effectively with people who have dementia demands highly developed interactive skills, which come naturally to some people but are difficult to teach. The rewards, however, in terms of mitigating distress and disturbance, can be significant. Speech and language therapists can provide helpful advice and guidance on minimizing the impact of dysphasia.

Box 4.1 Dysphasia

Expressive dysphasia

Involves difficulty saying what one wants to say, usually initially consisting of word-finding difficulties before progressing through to difficulties with sentence construction and maintaining conversational form.

Receptive dysphasia

Involves difficulties in understanding the verbal communications of others.

Countering the impact of dysphasia

Assisting understanding

Holding onto the notion of one's mother tongue becoming a foreign language can be helpful. If I am reasonably proficient in another language, but some way short of fluent, how do I need others to talk to me in order to maximize my understanding? I need them to talk:

- Clearly.
- Reasonably slowly.
- In manageable 'chunks' that I can 'translate' without getting behind in hearing what they are saying.

Equally, if someone needs to repeat something that I have not understood, it is better that they do so 'word-for-word' initially, before trying alternative words/phrases if I am still unable to make sense of it. In conversation I need to be allowed slightly longer than usual to form and articulate a response.

It is crucial to gauge the degree to which such measures are necessary in order to avoid either appearing unduly infantilizing on the one hand or 'outpacing' on the other. Find a balance—founded on observation and assessment—of encouraging the use of remaining skills without jeopardizing morale and self-esteem by setting up repeated experiences of failure.

Assisting expression

Sustaining interaction in the presence of expressive dysphasia requires a listener who is:

- Able to listen attentively and sensitively, using those words that are comprehensible in an attempt to 'fill out' what the person is trying to convey.
- Sensitive to the emotional tone behind the (attempted) words, who recognizes when failure is leading to exasperation and knows when it is time to stop.
- Prepared to engage imaginatively and creatively in conversations that may sound bizarre to others who are listening.

The social impact of dysphasia

As a general rule it is wise to assume that a person's understanding of language is less impaired than their ability to speak. Speaking about the person in the third person in their presence (the 'does he take sugar' syndrome) remains depressingly common in dementia care and should be avoided at any stage in the illness.

Non-verbal communication

Dysphasia will eventually rob the person with dementia of their ability to use and understand language, but it is important to keep in mind the role that non-verbal forms of communication play in the creation and maintenance of relationships and, therefore, in emotional well-being.

People with profound impairment of language skills can often judge with uncanny accuracy whether others are being friendly or aggressive, respectful or dismissive.

Responding to factually incorrect speech

Carers of people who are disorientated and still active face the challenge of spending sustained periods of time with someone whose understanding of their situation and surroundings differs radically from their own.

Given that the person with dementia will often want to act on the basis of that understanding, often in a way that may be harmful to their (and/or others') well-being, this poses real dilemmas for those involved in their care.

The natural response to factually incorrect speech content is to correct it. Sometimes, particularly in the earlier periods of the illness, this can be helpful. Often, however, it leads to resentment, frustration, conflict, and a sense of alienation, which exacerbates distress and disturbance.

Relationship is the key

Don't let factually inaccurate statements get in the way of building and maintaining a trusting relationship.

Utilize the relative strength of 'implicit memory' (📖 Box 6.3 p 148), which enables disorientated people to build relationships even in the presence of explicit memory problems. Carers can enhance the potential of their being perceived as a trusted friend and ally by:
• Appearing interested, concerned, warm, and supportive.
• Avoiding constantly correcting factually inaccurate speech.
• Demonstrating empathy by naming any negative emotions that the person appears to be experiencing.

Recreation

One of the most difficult challenges facing the carers of people with dementia is in meeting their need for recreation. From the childhood experience of 'playtime' at school through to adults pursuing hobbies, taking vacations, or enjoying various forms of entertainment, leisure time and relaxation form an important and pleasurable counterpoint to the world of work and productivity. It is an area in which individuals can exert control over how they utilize their time and resources. Many would argue that, alongside relationships, it is 'what makes life worth living'.

Selecting suitable activities

Advice and guidance from an occupational therapist with a good understanding of dementia can be very helpful here. Activities need to enable the person with dementia to experience:

- Engagement. Find out about their former interests, hobbies, and work. Try to get hold of items or artifacts that are related to their earlier lives. Be aware, however, that tastes and interests can change.
- Achievement. Take care not to draw attention to skills that have been lost by asking them to do things they used to be able to do but no longer can. Look for ways of making tasks easier—this can be done by:
  - Breaking tasks down into manageable chunks. It may be that planning a sequence of related tasks is too complicated, whereas each individual task is manageable in its own right.
  - Utilizing remaining skills. A woman with a well-retained knowledge of songs, for example, was given quiz questions where the answers were words from songs that the question master would sing the previous line of.
  - Making the level simpler.

As cognitive impairment progresses, an activity that in an earlier time was 'productive' can become a form of enjoyment. Relatively simple tasks such as dusting, for example, can become a pleasurable, sensory, repetitive experience.

Expressing sexuality

As with earlier life stages, in later life there continues to be a wide range of appetite for, and interest in, sexual activity. Whilst some people appear to find it less important, others continue to experience sexual desire and a need for physical intimacy that is scarcely diminished from their younger years.

Amongst the latter group, disorientation and declining social judgement may result in behaviour that brings alarm and anxiety to others. Whether this behaviour emerges within a pre-existing intimate relationship or with comparative strangers in a care setting, it requires sensitive and tactful handling.

In pre-existing relationships

Probably the most commonly encountered problem is that of a carer/partner of a person with dementia wanting less sexual contact than the person that they are caring for.

This could be the result of an increase in the desire of the person with dementia, brought about by factors such as forgetting when sexual activity last took place, boredom, or a perceived need to re-establish themselves as an equal within the relationship.

There may also be a diminution of interest in the carer. Dependency is, for all sorts of understandable reasons, somewhat inimical to sexual desire. One often witnesses a shift in the relationships between partners where one is becoming the carer of the other, who has dementia. This shift is towards a parent/child template, and its most overt indicator is the tone of voice that the carer begins to use towards the cared for. Within such a relationship, sexuality and physical intimacy can be experienced as taboo.

Where the imbalance involves a continuation of sexual appetite in the carer of someone who no longer shows any inclination towards sexual activity, complex issues regarding capacity to consent are raised. Carers commonly feel some degree of guilt and distress about continuing sexual relations when their partner's willingness to do so appears vague or compromised.

In care settings

Overtly sexual behaviour by people with moderate dementia in care settings is often categorized as 'challenging', indicating a perceived threat to the rights or well-being of others. Staff may also have difficulties in accepting the appropriateness of sexual desire in later life.

Where disorientation or disinhibition is leading to unacceptable displays of sexual behaviour in public spaces, such as masturbation or genital exposure, there is a need to balance the rights of other residents and staff not to have to witness such events with acknowledging an unmet need in the individual. Establishing that such sexual activity is not discouraged in private needs to be balanced with a policy of intervention when it is carried out in public.

Two people with dementia forming a new intimate relationship in a care setting raises a host of anxieties. If any form of sexual activity is involved then staff need to be able to ascertain whether both parties are giving meaningful consent. This will need to be considered in the light of prevailing law (📖 Chapter 11), although the law is a blunt instrument here.

If residents are deemed capable of being able to consent, then the impact on family relationships—possibly including a partner—will need to be addressed. Family members often tend to hold an exaggerated view of care facilities' powers to control the behaviour of their residents. Struggling with issues of loss and guilt, they may exert great pressure on staff to stamp out behaviour that they themselves are finding it difficult to bear.

When is sex not allowed?

Sexual activity is not allowed when one party is unable to refuse (the refusal is not necessarily verbal). Activity that is accepted (or unresisted) and takes place in a private house is almost certain not to be prosecuted. Objection or resistance would, of course, make sex illegal between two people with or without capacity.

Therefore:

• If the person with dementia appears distressed or unhappy, or is seen to resist advances and the sexual partner still has capacity, sex should be discussed with the partner. The partner should be informed that the activity does not appear to be a loving thing to do, and that it may be harmful and is probably illegal. This should prompt increased observation or review. If such discussion is ignored then action is required to protect the person with dementia. Alternatives might be suggested (the UK Alzheimer's Society has a helpful document at www.alzheimers.org.uk; click on About Dementia; Fact sheets; number 514 Physical intimacy).

- If both parties are cognitively impaired and lacking capacity they will still require protection; the above procedure should still be attempted although the participants may not be able to comprehend discussion.

Sleep

Sleeping problems are common amongst older people and some people with dementia have difficulty getting to sleep or wake through the night. Others seem to manage to sleep for much of the day and then all through the night. Persistent night-time disturbance is a burden for many carers and is often a major factor in deciding to seek placement in a care home.

In healthy elderly people, the total amount of time spent asleep does not change very much with ageing, but sleep is more broken with more episodes of waking during the night and more napping during the day. Elementary sleep hygiene procedures are the first line of treatment and are worth a try in people with dementia (📖 Box 4.2).

Simple measures

People with dementia frequently have disturbances in the normal day-night rhythms. These problems may be exacerbated by spending all day in the same place with the same carer. Attendance at a day centre where there are activities to keep the clients awake during the day sometimes helps to restore more normal circadian rhythms, although some day centre attenders are so exhausted by the day out that they fall asleep soon after returning home and then wake early the next morning. We have also found that respite care may be beneficial in getting patients' internal biological rhythms synchronized with day and night. The cues in a hospital or care home of the day staff leaving and night staff coming on duty, and the peer pressure of the other residents going to bed at the same time, are probably key elements in this.

Sleep rhythms are affected by levels of lighting. Quite high levels of illumination are required to promote daytime wakefulness and these are often difficult to achieve with artificial light. Daylight is a much more practicable source of strong light. Lack of adequate light causes people to fall asleep earlier each day, resulting in earlier wakening. Exposure to light helps to keep people awake until later in the evening and so maintain a more normal sleep pattern.

Box 4.2 Sleep hygiene

Environment:
- Ensure comfortable bedding and freedom from pain or physical discomfort.
- Room temperature should be cool, but not cold.
- Room should be well-ventilated with noise and light minimized.
- A small amount of lavender on a pillow can aid sleep.

Routine:
- Avoid sleep during the day.
- Establish a regular bedtime.
- Avoid caffeine, alcohol, spicy or sugary foods, and exercise for 4 h before going to bed. Try warm milk and a banana as a pre-bedtime snack.
- Take a warm bath before bed.

If unable to get off to sleep, or if you wake during the night and are unable to get back to sleep, leave the bedroom and read or sit quietly in low light until feeling ready to sleep.

Medication
- Many medicines may have an effect on sleep. In general it is advanta-geous to prescribe sedative agents to be given at bedtime, and those with a more alerting effect in the morning. Examples would include using sedative antipsychotic or antidepressant medications such as tra-zodone or risperidone at night to assist with sleep; and cholinesterase inhibitors such as donepezil and SSRI antidepressants like citalopram in the morning.
- Pruritus (itching) is a common symptom in older people, usually idi-opathic or as a result of dry skin. Look out for rashes and signs of scabies. A sedative antihistamine such as promethazine may help to relieve both itching and insomnia.
- Bear in mind that any sedative medication may increase unsteadiness and the risk of falling. This is not an absolute contra-indication to the use of sedating drugs, but always needs to be considered before pre-scribing.
- The BNF only recommends short-term use of hypnotic medications, although there is no definition of how long this period is. However, some people with dementia do seem to benefit from long-term treat-ment with hypnotics. If they are not experiencing adverse effects and their carers are enabled to continue to support them by this medica-tion, it will sometimes be in the best interests of the patient to con-tinue with long-term treatment.
- There is no clear first choice of a hypnotic agent. Clomethiazole (192mg to 384mg or 250 to 500mg clomethiazole edisilate syrup) has the advantage of a rapid onset of action and lack of hangover, but some people find the capsules difficult to swallow and the syrup tastes unpleasant. Also, it is sometimes ineffective. Alternatives are the 'Z' sleeping pills (zopiclone, zolpidem or zaleplon) or temazepam; other benzodiazepine hypnotics are best avoided because of the risk of daytime sedation or withdrawal reactions.

Problem behaviours

As dementia progresses, the capacity to make sense of one's environment and situation diminishes. We might, of course, expect that there will be a psychological reaction to this loss—perhaps a denial of what is happening, a barely contained sense of rage, or a regression to a child-like dependency on others and an inability to tolerate separation from attachment figures. The person with dementia also faces an ever increasing struggle to organize his or her actions in a way that ensures that his or her needs are met. This might include a number of fundamental needs, for things such as:

- Physical comfort.
- Occupation.
- Company.
- Stimulation.
- Self-esteem.
- Physical or psychological safety.
- Expression of sexuality.

If we add to this combustible mix an erosion of the ability to communicate successfully with others, along with the fact that individuals with dementia will tend, until the very late stages of the illness, to *do things*, to *act*, then we can begin to see that some degree of 'difficult behaviour', which brings distress to the person with dementia and/or to others, is bound to arise.

The assessment and management of behavioural difficulties in dementia presents the greatest of challenges to carers and to caring organizations. It is an emotionally charged area that is characterized by exasperation and frustration (often mixed with love and concern) felt by and towards the person with dementia. Clear thinking is at a premium in such an atmosphere and it can be difficult for those who are called in to assist to gain a clear and accurate understanding of exactly what is happening. Those involved often feel they have an urgent need to 'offload' the difficulties that they are facing.

The role of the professional is to:

- Acknowledge the strength of feeling.
- Introduce the capacity to think about:
  - what exactly is the problem behaviour?
  - what factors are bringing it about?
  - what potential ways are there of reducing the behaviour?
  - what actions might minimize its impact?

What is the problem behaviour?

The first thing that we need to get clear in our minds is exactly what the problem behaviour is. The plethora of labels commonly employed in this area can add to the confusion. Wandering, aggression, and shouting/screaming are the most commonly used terms, but they can hide as much as they describe.

We also need to assess who the behaviour is a problem for. The degree of distress that results from a particular behaviour will be partly determined by the behaviour itself and partly by the way in which others react. Some carers and care settings find relatively low levels of difficult behaviour and risk really difficult to bear and it might be that one focus for any intervention has to involve raising their toleration thresholds to a more realistic level.

It is also vital to pay attention early on to the extent of the problem. Ask caregivers to keep a diary for a few days that notes when the problem behaviour occurs, some indication of its intensity, and for how long it lasts. This can provide a 'baseline' against which the effectiveness of future interventions can be measured. Improvements can be difficult to discern in the daily busyness of care, and being able to demonstrate benefits can be crucial for caregivers to persevere.

What is causing the problem behaviour?

There are differing theories relating to the potential sources of difficult behaviour.

- The 'person-centred' school (⏚ Chapter 6 Box 6.6) tends to view difficult behaviours as a form of protest against the attack on person-hood that results from the 'malignant social psychology' surrounding dementia sufferers. They locate the problem in the attitudes and behaviours of caregivers and their impact on the person with dementia.
- A similar, but subtly different, claim to being a truly 'person-centred' approach has been pioneered by the psychologist Graham Stokes, who sees 'challenging behaviour' largely as the result of the 'unmet needs' of the person with dementia.
- Behavioural psychology employs a 'stimulus-response' model in an attempt to understand the factors that bring the behaviour about, utilizing the ABC approach (⏚ p. 157–8) in order to identify potential causes.
- More biologically orientated psychiatry tends to emphasize the role played by neuropathological damage in producing behavioural difficulties.
- Psychodynamically informed approaches emphasize the re-emergence of unresolved conflicts and the anxieties and distress that accompany the threat of psychic collapse.

Whilst the use of psychotropic medication is usually inappropriate before non-pharmacological interventions have been adequately explored, assessment does need to address whether the behaviour is symptomatic of a treatable mental health problem. Depression is under-diagnosed in people with dementia and psychosis can easily be missed when communication is severely impaired (⏚ p. 85). Physical causes of delirium or discomfort need to be considered, especially when the onset of the behaviour, or an increase in its intensity, is sudden.

It is also helpful to establish the previous patterns of behaviour of each individual. High levels of physical activity, a short temper, or a propensity to engage in physical violence may be lifelong characteristics that are simply continuing into the dementia.

What might reduce the problem behaviour?

Given the multiple origins of behavioural difficulties, it is only rarely that they will be completely eradicated. A more realistic aim is to reduce their frequency and intensity and to minimize their impact on others.

Caregivers should be encouraged to 'experiment' by trying out different approaches and measuring their impact. Wherever possible, members of a care team (either in a care home, or members of a family) should 'brainstorm' possible causes and then systematically try influencing them both individually and in combination.

Example 6.1

May, an 86-year-old resident with advanced dementia in the Havens Rest Home, is causing annoyance and distress to other residents by making a loud, shrill noise, sometimes for many hours at a time.

Hazel, her keyworker, and June, her daughter, have kept a 'noise' diary for a week and are looking at the results. They think one factor may be the amount of noise in the area of the lounge where May usually sits.

They decide to try sitting May for a few days in a quieter area, away from the TV and some of the more talkative residents. Firstly they try taking her there each time the 'shrilling' starts. Then they try taking her there before the shrilling begins—each time measuring how long it is before the noise begins again.

What might lessen the impact of the problem behaviour?

Given the modest success rates of both behavioural and pharmacological interventions in changing behaviour, a realistic approach pays much attention to managing the impact that the behaviour has on others. In communal care settings this might include ensuring that others have some time away from the company of the person displaying the unwanted behaviour. They may also need special measures to protect the safety of themselves and their property.

'Wandering'

What is the problem?

The term 'wandering' tends to be used to describe movement where the aim is not immediately obvious or which presents potential difficulties. The first question to ask is 'Is it a problem?' and if so, 'To whom?'.

If 'wandering' constitutes a seemingly contented resident who spends much of his or her time moving around a home in which most residents spend much of their time gazing towards a TV or napping, then perhaps he or she is the one *without* the problem. If, on the other hand, it describes somebody who has lost all traffic sense and is walking through the city centre at 3 a.m. in their nightclothes, then there is clearly an unacceptable level of risk.

Often it is not so much the movement that is the main source of concern as the way the person behaves as they move around. In residential homes this often includes entering the rooms of other residents and interfering with their possessions. The potential risks to self and to others and the infringement of their rights needs to be assessed.

What is causing the problem?

The person with dementia may not regard their walking as being purposeless. It is useful to establish what it is that they think they are doing.

Some wandering clearly contains an element of searching behaviour, as if the person is trying to find their way back to a situation in which they were more at peace. Attempting to seek out key figures, such as spouses or long-dead parents, may indicate that attachment needs are not being met in the current environment.

Familiar places, even the person's own home, can seem strange and alien, prompting an individual to set out in search of somewhere that feels like their 'real' home. This could be one aspect of a general sense of strangeness in which living in the world feels different, less predictable—perhaps reflecting the way in which the person's experience of their own mind is altered.

Akathisia from antipsychotic medication may be the primary cause of physical restlessness. Physical discomfort, such as pain experienced when sitting, or from constipation, can also make it difficult for someone to remain still.

What might reduce the problem?

Assistive technology, such as timer-set devices that trigger a voice message encouraging the person not to go out when an outside door is opened, may help those who are still living at home and who are putting themselves at risk by leaving the house at inappropriate times.

Sometimes family members, as a last resort, restrict the ability of someone with dementia to leave the home by making it difficult for them to get out, e.g. by locking the door. The balance of risks inherent in such a move (such as from fire, or injury trying to climb out of windows) needs to be weighed against the dangers people might face in going out. A move into residential care is often precipitated by family carers being unable to tolerate the anxiety provoked by a vulnerable family member who is repeatedly leaving the house and getting lost. Both families and care homes may employ key-code systems that require knowledge of a sequence of numbers or letters to unlock the outer doors. A similar 'key-safe' system allows those who know the code to access a key located on the outside of a family home in order to gain entry.

In residential settings, those who are constantly on the move may be encouraged to remain stationary by being engaged in some form of activity, although they may only be able to do so for brief periods. 'Little and often' may be the only feasible approach.

The Pool Activity Level (PAL) can assist in identifying activities that are appropriate to the individual, taking account of their cognitive and functional abilities. PAL combines life history information with a relatively easy to use observational assessment framework that identifies four activity levels to guide carers towards the suitable level of intervention with ADLs, as well as selecting activities most likely to meet recreational and occupational needs.

If levels of agitation are too high to allow sustained attention on a single activity, a person may respond to a substitute 'attachment figure' chosen from amongst the staff group. If such a staff member spends time unobtrusively accompanying the person with dementia on their 'search', and is able to become perceived as a potential companion, then they may in turn start to meet some of the attachment needs that are driving the constant searching. The ability to adopt such a role requires advanced interpersonal skills, time, and determination, and is emotionally demanding. There are training and organizational issues that will need to be addressed before such an approach can impact on behaviour.

Akathisia may respond to the withdrawal of neuroleptic medication but this can also, paradoxically, make the situation worse. Antimuscarinic drugs such as procyclidine and benzodiazepines such as lorazepam can help (but also risk making matters worse), as can a daily glass of red wine.

What might lessen the impact of the problem behaviour?
The person with dementia living at home and unable to give a coherent account of themselves should always have some form of identification about their person that others can access if they get lost. If the problem is persistent it can be worthwhile providing the local police with a photograph and description that can be used to alert officers when the person goes missing. Some families have set up discreet observations of one or more 'wanders' in order to check things such as:

• Where the person heads for.
• If they are able to make their way back.
• How safely they negotiate traffic.
• If, and how, they interact with strangers.

In residential settings, carers of people who are unable or unwilling to remain seated for any length of time find that attending to other care needs can be difficult. Maintaining adequate nutrition may require a creative use of finger foods that the person can eat whilst on the move. Physical access to the private areas and property of other residents may need to be restricted if somebody is moving into such areas and taking items in the belief that they are their own.

Aggression
What is the problem?
Aggression usually involves verbal or physical attack upon another person or their property. In dementia care it is most commonly associated with carers impeding the person with dementia from doing what they wish (such as leaving where they currently are to go 'home') or with carers doing things to the person with dementia that they do not want (most commonly personal care, such as cleaning after episodes of incontinence). In relation to aggression towards carers, therefore, it usually arises as a result of either frustration or fear. In residential settings it is not uncommon for people with dementia to behave with aggression towards each other; this usually has its origins in rivalry.

Health professionals called in to assist with aggression need to be aware that caregivers may feel the need to ensure that they do not underestimate the extent of the problem and will thus tend to over-compensate against this possibility by exaggeration. Unless the threat to bodily injury is serious and acute, getting some kind of realistic 'baseline' is desirable. Rather than asking a whole care team to keep a record it can be more productive to ask a willing individual to keep a diary of the aggressive behaviour over a week or so.

What is causing the problem?
Verbal and physical aggression are commonly reactions to fear or frustration. Impulse control can be impaired by dementia—particularly in relation to damage in the frontal lobes.

Whilst some people may always have been quick to resort to physical and/or verbal aggression, in dementia care it is most often the result of people working at cross-purposes. The greater the confusion and tendency to misinterpret the environment and the actions of others, then the greater the risk of aggression is.

What might reduce the problem?
Try to understand what is causing the behaviour that the carers need to inhibit. Fear can be lessened by reducing the potential for misinterpretation of actions and situations. Sensitive observation of verbal tone, facial expression, and body posture can usually provide warning signs of when a person is becoming alarmed and potentially aggressive. Avoid confrontation or acting in ways that are perceived as disrespectful (which commonly exacerbate potentially violent situations).

It is important to build up trust and rapport in relationships at times when people are not feeling threatened or aggressive. Personal care tasks that can be experienced as intrusive need clear and understandable explanations that are delivered in a calm and reassuring tone of voice. Careful notice should be taken of anything that makes such interventions more or less tolerable.

There will be occasions when it is wiser and safer to abandon planned care interventions and to try again later. There will also be occasions when the situation demands an immediate intervention (🕮 Chapter 6 p. 164).

Carers should always try to pay attention (and show that they are paying attention) to what the person with dementia is communicating—both verbally and non-verbally. It pays to try and see the situation as the person with dementia is seeing it, and to act accordingly to remove sources of anger, fear, and frustration. Coming alongside the person with dementia in an attempt to be perceived as a potential ally, rather than confronting them and being perceived as a threat or an obstacle, can serve to defuse many situations.

De-escalation techniques can enable carers to reduce the potential for anger developing into physical aggression. They involve the conscious management of verbal and non-verbal behaviour with the aim of reducing the level of anger in the person with dementia, and would include:
- Assuming a non-threatening body posture:
  - arms not raised or with hands on hips
  - shoulders not raised
  - not 'towering over'.

- Head leaning to one side or slightly down.
- Good, but not intrusive, eye contact.
- Respecting the person's personal space.
- Ensure they feel that they have an escape route.
- Approaching them only slowly and from the front.
- Reducing stimuli and obtrusive presence of others.
- Not contradicting or challenging what they are saying.
- Using a calming and reassuring tone of voice.
- Actively listening to what the angry person is saying.
- Acknowledging how they are feeling.
- Taking all the time that is necessary.

What might lessen the impact of the problem behaviour?

There will be occasions when the most sensitive and skilled interventions are unable to prevent incidents of verbal and physical aggression. Professional carers working with people who may become physically aggressive need to be trained in methods that maximize their own safety, as well as in the therapeutic use of physical interventions to manage aggression. In communal situations it is important to reassure other people present and assist them to do whatever is necessary to maintain their own safety.

Any episode of aggression requiring physical intervention should be followed by an opportunity for staff to debrief and evaluate the way in which the incident was managed. Good team work, with each member knowing their role in maximizing the safety of themselves, the person with dementia, and others is the ideal.

Aggression towards family carers is a common precipitant of the move into residential care. Advising family carers on de-escalation and on identifying potential causes of aggression needs to be coupled with advice on how to maintain their own safety. Although respite and day care can provide a much-needed break for family carers, sometimes such breaks are followed by an increase in hostilities, as the person with dementia seems to 'punish' their carer for the perceived abandonment.

Shouting and other persistent noises

What is the problem?

This is a problem that usually appears in the more advanced stages of dementia. It is particularly troublesome in communal living situations, where its impact on the mental well-being of others is most pronounced. With profoundly disabled people, making a noise and observing their surroundings can be amongst the few remaining things they are actually able to do without the help of others.

Again it is important to establish the nature and intensity of the behaviour:

- What is the noise like?
- Is it singing or conversational?
- Does it seem to indicate distress?
- When does it start and for how long does it carry on?

What is causing the problem?

In advanced dementia persistent vocalization that appears to indicate distress may be an expression of:
- Physical discomfort or pain(s).
- Psychosis (📖 p. 20).
- Anxiety or depression (📖 p. 18–20).
- Long-established patterns of behaviour.

Other commonly associated factors include:
- Social isolation.
- Poor quality interactions with carers.
- Boredom and lack of activity.
- Unintentional reinforcement from carers.
- Excessive stimulation.
- Compulsive repetition.

What might reduce the problem?

In advanced dementia communication difficulties can hinder the investigation of psychosis, depression, and physical pain or discomfort. Their detection and treatment can remove one or more of the major causes of persistent vocalization.

Carers should be encouraged to experiment with different approaches and to develop a systematic method of noting their impact on the nature, volume, and duration of noises. It is common, and natural, for carers and other residents to unintentionally reinforce vocalizations by reacting with admonitions or reassurance when they begin. If lack of social contact or boredom are factors then some investigation will be needed into activities and contacts that can serve as a source of pleasure. This might involve social contact, physical touch such as hand massage or grooming, sensory investigation of different materials, or the use of dolls or toys. Some care settings have employed 'artificial' contact, such as tape recordings or videos of family members.

It is important to introduce social contact when the desired outcome (i.e. quietness) is occurring rather than 'rewarding' the onset of persistent noisiness by input from carers. Initially this may exacerbate the 'protest' element of the behaviour, but over time systematic rewarding of the desired behaviour will yield results.

What might lessen the impact of the problem behaviour?

Ensuring that others are given some break from persistent noise can be essential to their well-being. Some form of physical separation will often be required. It is generally best to do this in a planned and systematic way, rather than resorting to physically removing someone from the communal environment at a point when everybody has 'had enough'; such moves can be perceived as, and descend into, punishment. Again, a period in which the noise is monitored and recorded can help to identify periods when it would be most appropriate for someone to spend time alone in their own room, for example.

Risk

'Risk' is a hazard, a chance of bad consequences or loss, or exposure to danger (*Concise Oxford Dictionary*).

Judging and taking risks for yourself is one of the privileges of adulthood. However, society limits or forbids some potentially risky behaviours, either:
- For the general good (traffic speed limits, industrial emission of pollution).
- To protect those who are powerless or vulnerable from the more powerful (industrial safety, child protection, care home regulations).

Inappropriately putting someone at risk, by act or omission, may be:
- Illegal under Health and Safety laws.
- Negligent (an abrogation of a duty of care).
- Unprofessional (not following guidelines or showing due concern).

Risk may be related primarily to health (injury, illness prevention), but may also be social (exploitation, mugging) or environmental (falls hazards in the home).

Risk is feared, both because of the possibility of undesirable outcomes, but also by staff because of the possibility of criticism, disciplinary action, litigation, or prosecution.

On the other hand, risk is never completely avoidable, and avoidance of risk carries a cost. Mainly this is through restrictions. These can be restrictions on what you do (driving a car, walking outdoors, going on holiday), where you live (private home or care home), or how much supervision or help you have. Many restrictions are self-imposed (for example not going out for fear of falling), but others are social (protectiveness of families or professional carers) or legal (not driving if not fit to do so). There may be costs if supervision, assistive technology, taxis, help, or care home residence are required.

Risk in dementia

There are two aspects to risk in dementia:
- Chances of adverse events is increased—falls or other injury, fire, getting lost.
- Judgement is impaired:
  - what risks to take
  - balance between legitimate ambition or objectives and any associated risks.

This is the familiar territory of decision-making, based on assessments of capacity or best interests (📖 Chapter 12). Risks (and other burdens) must be set against benefits. Inability to foresee risks or other consequences of a course of action may indicate lack of capacity. 'Best interests' does not necessarily mean avoiding all risk, however, but using currently and previously expressed wishes, values, and preferences, and those of people close to the patient, to inform a situation in which risks may be accepted or rejected.

Interestingly, in England and Wales, the Mental Capacity Act 2005 puts heavy emphasis on efforts to respect autonomy, perhaps as a corrective to the power imbalance that exists between professionals and vulnerable people with dementia and their families. But without explicitly saying so, it assumes that reasonably safe and practicable alternatives can be identified in a given situation, leaving much to (multidisciplinary) professional advice and judgement on what should actually be offered.

Managing risk

- Identify or anticipate risks. Decide who might be harmed and how. Risk may be to the person themselves, staff, other residents or patients, neighbours, or passers by. This requires thorough assessment, including history-taking about past behaviours and judgements, assessment of current physical and mental abilities, and consideration of the impact of different levels of help or environments (someone may perform better at home than in hospital; moving to a care home may increase risk by destabilizing or decompensating function).
- Acknowledge risk. Risks must be made explicit. There is no covering up—all too soon they will become apparent. Sometimes families will demand assurance that a situation is 'safe'. There is no alternative but to state that there is no such thing as 'totally safe', and that people with dementia live with greater risk than others.
- Minimize risk. Avoidable risks should be avoided if the cost in terms of restriction of function or choice is not compromised too much. This balance can only be decided in conversation and negotiation with the patient, those close to the patient, and other interested parties (health and social care professionals, care homes). The professional advisor must be neither too gloomy nor too optimistic, and must be sensitive to differences in perceptions of, and attitudes towards, risk.
- Reassess. Situations may have been misjudged or may change. Anticipated risks may or may not be borne out in practice, or new ones may emerge.
- Avoid blame. In risky situations, decisions made in good faith will sometimes go wrong. If things never go wrong it suggests lack of choice, too much restriction, and too conservative an attitude to risk. Looked at positively, a 'failure' represents new information. It has to be analysed to discover why it occurred, and the likelihood of its recurrence. It may be acceptable and desirable to take the same risk again, if that is what informed decision-making indicates. If things frequently go wrong, you must assure yourself that the gain (often respect for autonomy and freedom from restriction) has been worth the injury, upset, or inconvenience that results. However, you cannot set someone up to fail. You must identify when a liberal attitude becomes irresponsibility.

Quantifying risk

There is a tendency to think of risk in terms of life or death outcomes—breaking a hip, or falling under a bus. When something goes wrong, however, the outcome is more likely to be inconvenient than catastrophic. After a fall, for example, the chances of injury are 10%, of fracture 5%, and of hip fracture 1%. If someone wanders off and gets lost the chances are they will end up in a police station or hospital emergency department rather than in a traffic accident.

A key concept in risk assessment is to quantify:
- Probability of an outcome.
- Severity or desirability of the outcome.

A likely but trivial problem may be more acceptable than a rare but disastrous one.

Mitigating risk

The intervention will fit the problem, such as wandering, falls, malnutrition, physical aggression, or pressure sores.

One interesting area is the use of restraints to reduce risk. Restraint may be physical, chemical, or environmental. Preventing someone standing up from a chair may reduce the risk of falls, but is generally thought (in the UK at least) to be unacceptably restricting and compromising of dignity and 'personhood'. Some drug interventions may reduce the risk of aggression or agitation, but often cause as many problems as they solve.

A new variation on this is the use of electronic devices to signal risky behaviours or to allow tracking in the case of wandering ('tagging'). Examples include chair sensors that sound if the person gets up, or alarms on or near doors. These can alert staff to attend, or may act with a more 'behavioural' mechanism if the person automatically turns back from an alarmed entrance or sits down again to silence a chair sensor.

The use of these devices is controversial. On one hand they may increase freedom within limits (someone 'tagged' will be retrieved more quickly if they wander and get lost than someone not tagged) and allow staff to do more productive activities than constantly supervising and admonishing. On the other hand there is the suspicion that devices could be used to reduce employment of staff or make up for inadequate numbers.

Summary

1. In dementia, 'care' is the 'treatment'. 'Process' is more important than 'product'.
2. Caring for someone with dementia is demanding, and explicit carer support needs to be in place for both professional and family carers.
3. A balance must be drawn between promoting independence and avoiding failure. Interacting with someone with dementia in the wrong way makes things worse in terms of ability, behaviour, and quality of life.
4. There is a body of expertise in dealing with both activities of daily living and difficult behaviours that seeks to understand problems and needs, maximize involvement and abilities, and minimize use of sedative drugs.
5. Risk is increased in dementia. Risks should be identified, acknowledged, minimized, and reassessed.

Chapter 5

Dementia in the community

Services

The majority of people who receive a diagnosis of dementia are still living at home when this happens. As well as trying to appreciate the implications of what they have been told, people with dementia and their families must begin to find their way around a myriad of services. If they are successful in accessing these sources of help, it can make an enormous difference to their experiences in the years that lie ahead. Early involvement of people with dementia with a multidisciplinary community team has been shown to reduce problems as the disorder progresses. The availability and nature of services varies from country to country and region to region. Government policy is for everybody in the UK to have access to the services described in this chapter.

Care programme approach

People with suspected dementia may be seen in many different settings, by people from a wide range of professional backgrounds. Whoever sees the patient, in whatever setting, needs to consider the following outline of providing care:

- Assessment.
- Formulating a plan of care.
- Assigning a keyworker to ensure that the plan is implemented.
- Monitoring progress and reviewing and revising the care plan to ensure that it is still appropriate.

Assessment

- What does the person identified as in need of assistance see as the problem?
- What issues do family, friends and carers see as important?
- What is the background against which the problems have arisen?
  - past medical and psychiatric history
  - family and personal history
  - previous personality
  - home circumstances
  - activities and interests
  - support network.
- Current level of functioning.
- Medication.
- Risk assessment.

Care planning

- Is any change to the current care arrangements required?
- What additional services could help?
  - domiciliary care
  - day care
  - respite care
  - inpatient assessment
  - voluntary services: Age Concern, Alzheimer's Society etc.
- Are legal arrangements (Power of Attorney, Advanced Decisions, making a will, stopping driving etc.) necessary? See Chapter 11 and 12.
- Is the person entitled to financial benefits?
- Is a formal carer's assessment needed?
- Educational programmes.

Monitoring and reassessment

- Have services been provided?
- Are they working satisfactorily?
- Are additional resources required?
- Have the needs of the person with dementia or their carers changed?
- Is current medication satisfactory?
- Discuss with other agencies: are they are aware of other issues?

Community mental health teams (CMHTs)

What is a CMHT?

The mental health team is multi-professional and usually includes (in no particular order) nurses, doctors, a psychologist, and an occupational therapist. It may also include others, such as a physiotherapist, pharmacist, or social worker. In keeping with the major effort over the past 50 years to focus as much mental health care as possible in the community, these staff may work wholly or partly in the community (that is, outside hospital), seeing people at home, in care homes, or in locality health premises (hence the term 'community mental health team').

Most teams working for people with dementia have a primary focus on providing services for older people and also have expertise in dealing with 'functional' psychiatric disorders affecting older individuals. Younger people with dementia may have some difficulties accepting this focus (📖 Chapter 14).

Traditionally, mental health teams working with older people have taken on the care of anybody over 65 with a psychiatric disorder. This view is now seen as discriminatory and rigid age barriers are being removed; the focus of the older people's team is more on people who can benefit from their special expertise. This would include people with dementia of any age and younger people with functional illnesses who also have physical health issues. Team members can also offer advice on the management of comorbid psychiatric disorders to general hospital wards when patients from the team's area are admitted. Teams are nearly always associated with a consultant psychiatrist who also supervises the team's patients when they require inpatient psychiatric treatment.

Increasing specialization is becoming more normal and many teams have devolved responsibility for inpatients to specialist inpatient teams, particularly where the local population live some way from the admitting hospital. There are also now some dedicated teams for younger people with dementia, and liaison teams for older people in general hospital wards.

Common roles

All members of the CMHT work together to support people with dementia, their family and carers, and members of primary health and social care teams. Everyone has some responsibility for assessment, education, and treatment in their specific area of expertise; but they all need to develop an understanding of their colleagues' skills and limitations.

Every member of the team will deal with the person with dementia and undertake an assessment of problems, the likelihood of benefit from interventions, capacity to decide and best interests (📖 Chapters 11 and 12), and potential risks to the person and others who are caring for them. Anyone employed to provide care for other people has a duty of care to them.

In UK law this is summed up by the passage in Box 5.1.

Box 5.1 Duty of care

'You must take reasonable care to avoid the acts and omissions which you can reasonably foresee would be likely to injure your neighbour. Who then is my neighbour? The answer seems to be persons who are so closely and directly affected by my act that I ought reasonably to have them in contemplation as being so affected when I am directing my mind to the acts or omissions which are called in question.'

Donoghue v Stephenson [1932] AC 562

Members of CMHTs have a duty of care towards family members whom they are advising on the best way of dealing with a person with dementia who requires assistance.

Assessment

This will broadly follow the principles explained in Chapter 2.

Supporting

A degree of 'skills' transfer between the professional, family, and other carers might include sharing thoughts about the most helpful way to compensate for an individual's deficits without undermining remaining skills or self-esteem.

It may be possible to assist carers to develop strategies for minimizing (and surviving) changes in behaviour that cause distress and concern, by increasing understanding of the part that interpersonal and environmental factors can play in exacerbating such behaviour. This can help in maintaining people in their own homes and also in care homes.

People with dementia are often helped by a network of family, friends, and paid carers. It is necessary to assess informal aspects of the network—including the health and motivation of partners, family carers, friends, and neighbours—as well as formal support from statutory and voluntary sectors, such as home care services, meals at home, day care, and respite care facilities.

Other professionals

Team members can develop close relationships with primary health and social care teams to educate and support them in matters relating to dementia. They can also link to their colleagues in services for working age adults and can advise on transfers between teams.

Advocacy

Team members should act as advocates for people who are not able to mobilize support for themselves, although in some circumstances people with dementia and their carers will require specialist advocacy, independent of services.

Members of the team can act as familiar faces to ease the transition into day care or respite care, or during hospital admissions.

Specific roles
Community psychiatric nurses
Community psychiatric nurses (CPNs) are usually the largest group in a community mental health service for people with dementia. Their role will vary according to local arrangements and the availability and skills of other professionals; their training enables CPNs to work very flexibly. They are often well placed to respond to emergencies and can deliver urgent care, sometimes after discussions with members of other disciplines. Individual CPNs are able to develop specialist expertise by working with a specific client group, or in a restricted geographical area, or with certain other professionals.

Mental health
CPNs are well placed to assess the impact of the experience of dementia on an individual's mental health. They need the knowledge and expertise to identify the presence of psychoses, depression, or anxiety states within the context of a dementing illness. With recent changes to the Mental Health Act in England and Wales, CPNs can now take on the role of Approved Clinician or Approved Mental Health Professional and participate in decisions on enforced detention and treatment.

Treatment
Nurses, and particularly CPNs, are increasingly able to take on the primary role in treatment. They may develop skills in psychological therapies such as interpersonal therapy and cognitive-behavioural therapy or in prescribing of medication.

Occupational therapists (OTs)
An OT who is part of the CMHT will usually be better placed than their colleagues in Social Services or Primary Care to meet the needs of the person with dementia who is living at home. Their experience in working in dementia care is important in relation to a number of areas.

Physical aids and adaptations
The successful provision of aids and adaptations to help compensate for physical disabilities requires an understanding of the implications of cognitive impairment. In addition to assessing which aids may be the most helpful, the CMHT OT should be able to judge whether the individual with dementia can use it effectively.

The role of assistive technology that compensates directly for particular cognitive deficits has increased. Many sensors and remote control devices are now available, and more will soon be introduced. The presence of flood, carbon monoxide, and smoke detectors may reduce the risk of people with dementia inadvertently bringing harm to themselves or their neighbours. The assessment of this technology requires specific expertise in order to identify the most appropriate aids to promote independence.

People with impaired mobility may be unable to reach the door to allow in social or health care professionals. A key safe—a digital-lock protected external repository for house keys—can help overcome this. An 'entry-phone' intercom with electronic door opening is an alternative.

Summoning help in an emergency—for example after a fall—can be facilitated by using a pendant alarm. Designed to be worn around the neck, the alarm system uses the telephone to alert a call centre, who can call back or alert relatives or emergency services if the alarm is activated. Systems may be built in (cord alarms) in sheltered accommodation, where a warden may be on hand to help. This only works if the alarm is worn, can be operated, and is not overused, for example by repeated non-emergency calls for help.

Activity

CMHT OTs are able to provide advice on techniques and strategies for maximizing independent functioning at home, both to the person with dementia themselves and to family and other carers. This might involve reorganizing daily living routines and finding ways to enable the maintenance of social and leisure activities.

Working with family members

Maximizing the independent functioning of individuals with dementia often involves delicate and sensitive negotiation with partners or other close family members. Some partners find it difficult to tolerate the anxiety of seeing the person with dementia perform tasks less successfully than they have in the past, and move to 'take over' such tasks, leaving their partner to lose skills more rapidly. Carers for their part may have severely limited opportunities for activities outside the home. Working with family carers to reverse these trends requires an ability to contain the anxieties of family members, an ability that is more commonly found in professionals who have had experience in working in the field of mental health.

Risk assessment

The ability to contain anxiety is also helpful in situations where it is necessary to assess the feasibility of a person with dementia continuing to live alone at home. Families vary greatly in their capacity to tolerate the risks inherent in a person with dementia living alone; some come to the conclusion that some form of residential care is required before the individual with dementia does, while others seem oblivious to real dangers (📖 Chapter 4 p. 102).

When the OT's role is to support the person with dementia's desire to continue living at home, and to initiate the necessary measures to enable them to do so, then the working alliance with family members can be put under great strain. Awareness of family dynamics and an ability to reflect and adapt relationships in the light of these are skills that OTs in specialist mental health teams are able to develop.

Assessment of functioning

Assessment of functional abilities (extending beyond maintaining independence and meeting occupational needs) forms a key part of the overall assessment process. Specific tools such as MEAMS and Large Allen Cognitive Levels (LACL) (📖 Chapter 13 p. 324), as well as baseline functional assessments, can be important contributors to the decision-making processes around prescription of anti-dementia medications and other aspects of care management.

Physiotherapists

People with dementia may not be able to benefit from traditional physiotherapy that relies upon their co-operation with a regime of exercise and activity between sessions. They are at greater risk of falls than other older people and they have a greater incidence of cerebrovascular disease and features of Parkinsonism.

The physiotherapist working with people with dementia requires appropriate communication skills and the ability to make creative use of available resources. This may involve training carers to remind the person with dementia to do the appropriate exercises at the appropriate time. It is also likely to be relatively labour intensive, requiring frequent one-to-one interventions for a time-limited period. Although this may seem expensive, it is worth remembering that declining mobility is often a deciding factor in precipitating transfer into residential care.

Physiotherapists can advise informal carers about taking care of their own health and safety needs when assisting the person with dementia to mobilize or to transfer. Such carers are often performing manual handling tasks within the home that would not be attempted in formal care environments without support from colleagues or specialist equipment.

Social workers

There are a number of different management arrangements for collaboration between social work and community mental health services in different localities, making it difficult to make general statements about the role of the social worker. The social worker will often play a key role in both mobilizing the necessary support to enable people with dementia to stay at home and, when this is no longer feasible or desirable, in making the transition to residential care.

The social worker will be working with people with dementia and their carers at a point where difficult, often very painful, decisions are being made. They provide support and practical advice whilst balancing the rights of all parties and being mindful of the risks inherent in any chosen course of action.

Psychologists

Clinical psychology is the application of psychology to mental illness or mental health problems. All clinical psychologists will have completed a first degree in psychology and then received a broad clinical training before specializing in a particular area.

Within the dementia team the clinical psychologist will have a variety of roles. Many will be able to offer a detailed neuropsychological assessment in order to clarify the presence of a cognitive impairment and the nature of that problem based on the profile of deficits. Clinical psychologists may also conduct functional analyses of behaviour, which can be particularly useful in more advanced cases of dementia where spoken communication is compromised. Results from such assessments can be useful for other professionals and care providers in helping formulate care plans and the management of problematic behaviour.

Psychologists are increasingly involved in cognitive rehabilitation and may work closely with occupational therapists. Their broader role will include offering psychological interventions for mental health problems and this can have an application to dementia both in terms of working with individuals who are adjusting to the diagnosis and with individual carers and family members.

Many clinical psychologists work as a supervisory and consultative resource for other members of the CMHT and inpatient units, as well as seeing patients in their own right.

Speech and language therapists

Access to speech and language therapists (SALTs) is relatively new to many community mental health services and their potential contribution to the treatment of language difficulties in dementia remains relatively unexplored.

SALTs contribution to the assessment and management of swallowing difficulties (dysphagia) is more established, although this is often restricted to inpatient and residential services where the majority of such need is found due to its tendency to appear in the later stages of dementia.

Memory services

What is a memory clinic?

The term memory clinic has been used to describe a variety of activities. The term was first commonly used in the 1970s in North America to describe clinics that were essentially academic in their activities; their primary aim was to recruit people for clinical trials of anti-dementia drugs. By the early 1980s they began to arrive in the UK, and these clinics typically had a greater focus on service delivery. Dementia is the main focus of most memory clinics and the name appears to have arisen in an effort to avoid the stigma of specific conditions such as Alzheimer's disease. They are more easily defined by their activity than by their component parts, although the pattern of skills available in a clinic has implications both for the type and level of assessment offered and for subsequent interventions. Diagnosis, prescription, and monitoring of medication are the goals of most memory clinics. A potential negative consequence of this is that services geared to prescription may exclude those who are not suitable for medication.

Memory clinics assess, evaluate, and treat problems that present with cognitive impairment and behavioural change. Consequently memory impairment may be the most common subjective complaint of those attending but is typically only one of a number of presenting features.

Most memory clinics are multidisciplinary and their skill mix will reflect both the purpose and philosophy of the clinic and what it offers.

In the broadest sense, memory clinics attempt to:
- Accurately diagnose a dementia as early as possible.
- Initiate medical, psychological, and social treatment at the earliest opportunity.
- Monitor any interventions.
- Provide education, help, and support for clients and carers.
- Have a more general role in improving the quality of dementia care.

The component parts of a memory clinic vary but typically they are led by old-age psychiatrists, geriatricians, or neurologists. The team usually comprises:
- Psychiatric nurses.
- Occupational therapists.
- Clinical psychologists or neuropsychologists.
- Social workers.

Clinics may aim to work as 'one stop shops' with patients seeing professionals from several disciplines at one visit, but sometimes they may more closely resemble a 'virtual' team, with investigations being requested from OT and Psychology in the same way that more physiological measures such as blood tests and CT scans would be ordered.

In some areas a single community dementia team operates their own clinic; some memory clinics relate to a number of community teams.

The range of interventions offered by a memory clinic or service can be very broad and include:
- Diagnosis.
- Baseline assessment and further monitoring pending a diagnosis.
- The prescription and monitoring of pharmacological treatments specifically for dementia.
- The prescription and monitoring of other psychotropic medications to help people manage the problems associated with dementia.
- Advice regarding compensatory strategies to manage the consequences of cognitive impairment. These may include assistive technologies, cognitive rehabilitation etc.
- Behavioural interventions.
- Education and support at point of diagnosis.
- Continuing education and support for carers.
- Signposting of other resources available from other providers such as the voluntary sector and social services.

Advantages of memory clinics
- A concentration of expertise and a single point of access.
- Continuity.
- The availability of a variety of interventions.
- A multidisciplinary resource.

Disadvantages of memory clinics
- Large regional variations.
- Some clinics only offer medication and therefore provide no service to other individuals with cognitive impairment.
- How long should the clinic remain involved with an individual case? Carers may still appreciate support and information but clinic attendance may not appear to benefit the client to any degree.
- The problem of 'MCI' (📖 Chapter 1 p. 12). Should the clinic continue to monitor and if so for how long?
- GP referral rates may be low due to a lack of awareness or understanding of what the clinic can offer.
- Some individuals may be resistant to attending the clinic and require a more community orientated intervention.
- Those clinics established as prescribing services must alter their activities in line with prescribing guidelines.

Day care

The availability of day care for people with dementia is dependent upon location but where it is accessible and well-organized it has the potential to form a key part of the 'network of care' that can help support a person remaining in their own home.

Introducing day care

Entering an unfamiliar social situation, without the support of a partner or other key attachment figure, can be an overwhelming experience for many people with (or without) cognitive impairment. Accepting an offer of day care may feel to both carer and cared-for like the start of a 'slippery slope' that will lead inexorably to long-term residential care. This risks provoking feelings of guilt in the carer and abandonment in the person with dementia.

With these realities in mind, it is usually wise to:

- Introduce the idea gradually—encourage the person and their carer to make a short visit to be introduced to staff and other attenders before thinking of staying for a full day.
- Ask the person to attempt a trial day, with no commitments on either side. They can then come once 'with nothing to lose'.
- Ensure attachment needs are met. A person may need to attend with a familiar carer on the first day.
- Nominate a member of staff to meet and greet the newcomer and devote some time to developing rapport.
- Encourage the carer to 'pop out', initially for brief periods, then for longer spells as tolerated.
- Be flexible about transport arrangements and length of day. Many people are not willing or able initially to get on the day centre transport and to remain at the centre without distress for a full day.

Pros and cons of day care

In the earlier and middle stages of dementia good quality day care can provide:

- Social contact.
- Opportunity to utilize remaining skills.
- Stimulation.
- A structure to the day.
- Improved sleep.
- Respite for carers.

We have to acknowledge that there are also those for whom the carer respite function is paramount. Whilst day care may be of little or no direct benefit to the immediate well-being of the person with dementia, it is sometimes crucial to enabling them to continue living at home.

Box 5.2 Potential problems with day care

Day care can be a daunting prospect. It is depressing how readily some services are prepared to upset new attenders who are in the earlier stages of dementia.

Receiving a diagnosis of dementia often raises a host of anxieties about a future characterized by loss, humiliation, abandonment, and fragmentation. To take someone who is trying to keep a full awareness of these realities at bay and sit them amongst a group of people who are much more seriously impaired by illness than themselves might almost be construed as a form of psychological torture.

If day care becomes intolerable (☐ Box 5.2), alternative forms of respite must be sought. In some areas 'sitting services' are available, involving regular visits by a trained 'sitter' who cares for the person in their own home, enabling the family carer to go out. Befriending schemes involve volunteers visiting and taking the person out—often invaluable sources of support to older, less mobile carers with partners with dementia who still love to walk!

Residential respite care

Many people with dementia who are living with family carers will go for short periods, usually 1–2 weeks, into a care home or hospital unit in order to allow their family a break from caring or to enable them to get away on holiday.

Whilst such breaks may be disorientating and somewhat distressing for the person with dementia, this can be justified by the hope that they will be able to remain at home longer if their carer's needs for respite are met and they can avoid 'burn out'. It may also facilitate a future move into longer-term care. Having said that, carers occasionally find the prospect of returning to providing 24 hour care intolerable after they have experienced a break.

If respite care is used, it is best to find a residential or nursing home that can be used consistently, where staff have the opportunity to become familiar with the person's needs over a number of admissions. If there is a possibility of this being in the same facility that they attend for day care then so much the better. However, it is usually not a good idea for them to attend day care during their admission, as problems can arise at the end of the day when everyone else is going home and the person with dementia cannot remember or understand why they are being asked to stay.

Respite care can also be an opportunity to test out an individual's reaction to staying in a residential or nursing home environment and to discover the type of environment that is best suited to each individual. There is often a price to be paid, however, in terms of increased disorientation—as a tenuous grip on managing in a familiar environment is disrupted—or of anger towards family members for perceived abandonment. If care facilities are able to be flexible, it can help for periods of respite to start short and then be gradually lengthened. If the degree of distress and disorientation seems to be too great a price to pay then other methods of providing the carer with a break need to be explored.

Admission to a psychogeriatric ward

The specification of most old-age psychiatry services includes a 'dementia assessment ward'. It will be clear that in contemporary practice most assessment takes place in the community. Nevertheless there is still a vital role for inpatient assessment in a few cases, although this is now used much more sparingly.

Indications for admission to hospital:
- Assessment under the Mental Health Act (📖 Chapter 11).
- Breakdown of a complex care package.
- Sudden behaviour change or psychosis without obvious physical illness, making home care difficult.
- Transfer from an acute medical ward of people with previously unknown dementia who cannot immediately be discharged, where behaviour or psychosis is making management difficult on a non-specialist ward.

Home care

Help with personal and domestic activities is often a key factor in sustaining individuals with dementia who are living at home—especially those who are living alone. In addition to the valuable practical assistance provided, for many it is the primary source of social contact with the outside world. Home care that is flexible enough to work with the unpredictable habits and behaviours of people with dementia will fulfil this function more effectively than that which dictates that its workers must operate within tightly bound time limits and perform a prescribed list of chores.

Supporting carers

Definitions

There are a number of different definitions of 'carer', and each one provides a different set of challenges.

Paid

Professional carers will have a variety of backgrounds, training, and access to supervision. It is ironic that those who spend the most time in direct contact with people with dementia will typically be those who have the least access to training and support.

A professional role insulates paid carers from the emotional impact of caring for a family member, but typically carers will develop relationships with people with dementia over a period of time and can find themselves experiencing a high degree of distress as they see people with dementia develop greater levels of impairment.

Approaches such as person-centred care (📖 Chapter 4) seek to limit the negative impact of some of the common problems in care environments. Carers may depersonalize individuals to a certain extent, as a defence against the pain of seeing them deteriorate. In addition, performing intimate physical care upon people can be psychologically difficult and a certain professional distance can feel helpful to a paid carer and to the person receiving care.

In any caring occupation, access to good quality training and supervision is of paramount importance.

Unpaid/family/informal

Identification as a carer is a matter of definition and can be ethically problematic (📖 Box 5.3).

Box 5.3 Who is a carer?

The term carer (or caregiver) is loose and variably-defined. Organizations representing unpaid carers (sometimes called 'informal carers') often seek to draw a distinction from paid ('statutory' or 'professional') carers.

Definition: 'Someone who looks after a partner, relative, or friend, because of illness, disability, frailty, or the effects of old age.'

An alternative definition captures the idea of burden imposed by caring responsibilities: 'Someone whose life is in some way restricted by the need to be responsible for the care of someone who is mentally ill, mentally handicapped, physically disabled or whose health is impaired by sickness or old age.' (Pitkeathley: *It's my duty isn't it?* London, Souvenir Press, 1989.)

Some carers provide direct physical care, sometimes very intensive and intimate, some provide intermittent help with more difficult tasks (e.g. bills, shopping, household maintenance), and others may provide emotional support, advocacy, oversight, or help arranging support.

Difficult questions include:
- Who decides you are a carer and when do you cease to be a carer?
- What is normal 'helping' (e.g. sharing jobs within a family) and what is special 'caring'?
- Are you still a carer if your relative is placed in residential or nursing care?
- How long after the death of a relative do you cease to be a carer?
- Are you legally defined as a carer by health and social services? (In the UK carers are entitled to an assessment of their own needs, and may be paid benefits depending on the amount of time spent caring and the entitlement to benefits of the person receiving care.)

Patterns of carers' stress

Several different sources of stress have been identified in the literature:

- Identity: The problems of changing from a partner or child into a carer.
- Intra-psychic strains: The impact of caring upon self-esteem and loss of self.
- Bereavement: Individuals typically describe a process of ongoing bereavement where they see their loved one gradually disappearing. In addition many people grieve the loss of a future they had been looking forward to. Retirement plans rarely include looking after an incapacitated partner and people may find themselves very angry about the injustice of what they have lost.
- Physical resources: The practical and financial resources available to the individual.
- Social resources: The family and social networks available to the individual.
- Psychological resources: The individual's personality and psychological coping mechanisms.

Patterns of carer stress identified in the research literature:

- Carers' ratings of disability and of disturbed behaviour are the strongest predictors for carer well-being. This is stronger than relationship or socio-demographic variables.
- Depression in the carer is associated with low mood and disturbed behaviour in the person with dementia.
- Low levels of social support relate strongly to depression.
- Loss of companionship through diminished quality of communication.
- Loss of reciprocity due to increased dependency and deterioration in social behaviour.
- Carer satisfaction comes from continued reciprocity, mutual affection, companionship, job satisfaction, and fulfilment of sense of duty.

Box 5.4 Gender differences

Men and women have been found to differ in their response to social support.

Men tended to feel grateful for any input from domiciliary services and were relieved of some of their stress.

Women tended to feel guilty about needing to rely on outside help, which made them feel inadequate.

Factors making caring more potentially stressful
- Carer living with care recipient.
- Having a closer relationship with care recipient.
- Greater extrinsic motivators to care (feeling that one has been pressured into caring) and poorer quality of relationship. (Conversely those with more intrinsic motivators such as admiration and a better relationship experienced lower levels of stress.)
- Carer's perception of external pressures such as guilt, duty, responsibility.
- Difficulty getting away on holiday.
- Social life being affected.
- Household routines upset.
- Interrupted sleep.
- Cultural issues (these remain relatively under-researched).

Three types of intervention can be identified:
- Education on:
  - the nature of different dementias
  - coping strategies
  - specific approaches such as behavioural management
  - services available in different localities.
- Peer support.
- Therapy: formal psychological therapy following a specific model.

These interventions tend to be cumulative, with therapy containing a large educational component as well as peer support. Although group interventions are common, interventions can also be delivered remotely (e.g. from written materials) or on an individual basis.

Although research on carers remains limited, some studies have made interesting observations that appear counter-intuitive.
- One study reported that attendance at a day centre by the person with dementia did not alleviate carers' stress.
- A different study showed increased knowledge of dementia led to lower levels of depression but higher anxiety. However, carers felt more confident and competent as caregivers.
- A further study showed that key factors associated with decreased carer stress were frequency of CPN visits and day care. It also identified faecal incontinence and inability to communicate at any level as additional stressors.

Elder abuse

The most contentious area in health and social care for many years has been the protection of vulnerable children. Paediatricians and social workers have been faced with impossible dilemmas and have been subject to vilification whatever action they have taken to try to protect children. People with dementia are equally vulnerable, and abuse is regrettably common in hospitals, care homes, and in the community. (For abuse in care homes 📖 Chapter 7 p. 183.)

The charity Action on Elder Abuse defines abuse as: 'A single or repeated act or lack of appropriate action, occurring within any relationship where there is an expectation of trust, which causes harm or distress to an older person.' It covers a spectrum of behaviour with clearly criminal acts at one end (assault, fraud etc.) and poor standards of care, or neglect, at the other.

Many organizations have a role in preventing, detecting, and monitoring abuse. All prospective employees and volunteers need to be checked by the Criminal Records Bureau and under Protection of Vulnerable Adults procedures before they are taken on. Care workers who have harmed a vulnerable adult or placed a vulnerable adult at risk of harm (whether or not in the course of their employment) are banned from working in a care position with vulnerable adults. Anyone who employs a care worker is bound to report the employee if they are guilty of misconduct that has harmed or placed at risk a vulnerable adult. The Mental Capacity Act has introduced a new offence in England and Wales, of abusing or wilfully neglecting a person without capacity.

Abuse occurs within relationships. There are different pressures on informal carers—who are likely to have shared their lives with the person for whom they are willingly caring without pay—and those who are employed to attend to a person who needs care, and should themselves be under supervision (see Box 5.5). However, it is clear that stress in paid and unpaid carers predisposes them to abuse, and supporting them can help to mitigate the worst consequences. Education about the nature of dementia and how to communicate best with people with dementia can be of great benefit.

Box 5.5 Causes of elder abuse

For those living at home, predictors of abuse include:
- Poor quality long-term relationships.
- Carer's inability to provide the level of care required.
- Pattern of family violence exists or has existed in the past.
- Carer with mental or physical health problems.
- Social isolation of the family member.

The Alzheimer's Society observes that 'Caring for a person with dementia is often very demanding. People with dementia sometimes behave in ways that seem aggressive or violent as they try to deal with their experience of dementia, which could involve high levels of stress, frustration, and fear. This behaviour can be highly stressful for carers and highly predictive of mistreatment and abuse. There is ample evidence that carer and care worker stress is related to levels of support. Greater understanding about the disease process and ways of working with people with dementia can help—for example improved communication skills.'

Detecting abuse

A list of signs that should alert you to the possibility that abuse may be occurring is given in Box 5.6. But note that none of these is specific to abuse and all may have perfectly innocent explanations.

Box 5.6 Warning signs of possible abuse

Physical:
- Unexplained injuries, especially lesions on the face, torso, back, buttocks, or thighs.
- Clusters of injuries.
- Injuries at different stages of healing.
- Misuse of medication—e.g. excessive use of sedation.

Sexual:
- Difficulty sitting, change in gait.
- Perineal lesions.
- Rectal or vaginal bruising or bleeding (NB piles and carcinoma of the rectum are more common).

Psychological:
- Unexplained anxiety and distress.
- Passivity and resignation.

Financial:
- Sudden inability to pay bills or maintain lifestyle.
- Inappropriate financial transactions.

How to respond to suspected abuse

If you suspect a member of the victim's family or an informal carer to be abusing an adult who lacks capacity, you should follow local procedures to deal with this. In the UK, local authorities are required to have policies in place to investigate and manage suspected cases of abuse; Social Services usually act as lead agency for these procedures (often referred to as 'Vulnerable Adults Policies'). In England and Wales an Independent Mental Capacity Advocate (📖 Chapter 11) may be needed to safeguard the victim's interests.

Where individuals are at risk of financial abuse it will probably be necessary to involve the Office of the Public Guardian; the Court of Protection (📖 Chapter 11) may appoint a deputy to manage the affairs of the person who lacks capacity. It may be difficult to get formal arrangements in place for a person who is able to write cheques or withdraw cash from a bank, but who can be persuaded to spend their money irresponsibly. At present the emphasis in the British legal system is more on preserving the liberty of people to make foolish or imprudent decisions than on protecting the assets of people with impaired capacity.

Box 5.7

Good arrangements for the protection of vulnerable adults will ensure effective liaison between health professionals, social care workers, the police, and welfare benefits agencies. One agency, usually Social Services, will have been nominated to take the lead role.

Neglect, abuse or inadequate care?

At one end of the spectrum referred to earlier, in which the health and well-being of the person with dementia is in serious jeopardy, there can be no alternative to reporting suspicions immediately—possibly involving the police—and ensuring that the person has care provided within a place of safety.

In many instances, concerns over the well-being of the person with dementia are prompted by family carers who are lacking (some combination of) the physical, emotional, and material resources required to provide adequate care.

In such circumstances there needs to be discussion about whether it is in the best interests of the person with dementia to continue to be cared for at home. If it is, then every effort should be made to enhance those resources—thus reducing the potential for neglect or abuse. This may involve additional support at home, breaks for the carer, and increased psychological support. Careful monitoring will be required to ensure that the person with dementia is not put at unacceptable risk.

Professionals need to ensure that their collective anxieties about accepting uncertainty and risk do not overwhelm consideration of the person with dementia's right to remain in an emotionally supportive long-term relationship.

A note of caution

Signs of abuse, particularly where the principal carer is the perpetrator, should not automatically be taken to imply that the victim needs to be removed to a place of safety. People with dementia can generate huge levels of stress in their carers and are often verbally and physically abusive themselves; it is not surprising if on occasions the carers are unable to resist the temptation to retaliate. The benefits for a person with dementia of being looked after by someone with whom they have a long-term emotional relationship may be considerable and it may be appropriate for the carer to be supported rather than condemned. Removing the need for the principal supporter to provide intimate physical care may be enough to maintain a good emotional relationship.

Driving

Of all the skills acquired by young people, the ability to drive a car is most highly valued. It becomes an essential aspect of life in middle age, and as physical frailty ensues with ageing it plays an even more central role as alternative means of maintaining mobility and independence become less feasible.

It is small wonder that any suggestion that older people should stop driving is often met with fierce resistance.

Ageing motorists are likely to have more accidents than people of 21–65, but still have fewer than teenagers. This trend is exaggerated by some commonly used accident statistics. Accident rates are often expressed in terms of the accidents per number of miles driven, and older car-users drive shorter distances. They also drive mostly on roads around their homes, which are likely to be used by children, pedestrians, and cyclists. It is on these roads that the majority of accidents occur.

Cognitive impairment is only one factor that increases the hazards of motoring for older people. Sensory impairment, particularly poor eyesight, is a much greater risk. Equally important is decreased mobility, especially a reduced range of movement in the neck, which prevents the driver being able to look to the left and right and into rear view mirrors. Other factors such as impaired judgement and slower reaction times are also important.

Insight into driving ability is a key factor to be considered. If people with mild dementia are aware of their limitations and adapt their driving accordingly they may be safe to carry on. Many older drivers will not drive at night or in bad weather and will only go out with a passenger who can help and reassure them. Those who attempt to drive long distances when tired or who attempt unfamiliar routes alone are less likely to manage their vehicles safely.

In the UK the DVLA requires drivers over 70 to reapply for a licence each year. In the forms an applicant is asked to declare any medical condition that affects them. Where an applicant reports a neurological condition the DVLA approach the applicant's doctor with a NEURO2C form. This also contains questions about matters such as epilepsy and stroke. The questions in relation to cognitive impairment are shown in Box 5.8.

The DVLA manual for doctors ('At a glance standards of fitness to drive' www.dvla.gov.uk) states:

'It is extremely difficult to assess driving ability in those with dementia. Those who have poor short-term memory, disorientation, lack of insight and judgement are almost certainly not fit to drive.

'The variable presentations and rates of progression are acknowledged. Disorders of attention will also cause impairment. A decision regarding fitness to drive is usually based on medical reports.

'In early dementia when sufficient skills are retained and progression is slow, a licence may be issued subject to annual review. A formal driving assessment may be necessary.

'In every case where the diagnosis of dementia is clear, the person with dementia should be told to declare this condition to the DVLA.'

Box 5.8 Assessing fitness to drive

4. Is there evidence of cognitive impairment?
If yes, is there:
a) *Significant* impairment of behaviour sufficient to cause disorientation?
b) *Significant* loss of judgement?
c) Inappropriate behaviour?
If yes, please give brief details.
5. Is there currently sensory inattention?

If family or friends give a clear account of potentially hazardous driving, then the person with dementia should be advised to stop driving. If there is doubt about the ability to drive, or if the person with dementia is reluctant to accept advice, formal driving assessments can be arranged (for a fee) at specialist disabled drivers assessment centres. Neuropsychological assessment using tools such as the SDSA (📖 Chapter 13 p. 334) may help identify people who require a driving test.

If people with dementia continue to drive when this is unsafe, then it is the health professional's duty to notify the DVLA. Such action, even if theoretically a breach of confidentiality, is justified because of the risk to other people. Some thought should be given as to which member of the health care team should make the notification; in general it is best for the team leader to take on this responsibility to try to maintain the relationship between the keyworker and the person with dementia.

Holidays

Families are often first made fully aware of the extent of a person's cognitive difficulties when they get repeatedly lost or disturbed whilst away on holiday. Being removed from familiar, well-learned surroundings can expose the true extent of deficits and result in insurmountable obstacles to learning about and adapting to a new environment.

When planning holidays, therefore, it is important to keep in mind that the greater the unfamiliarity of the environment, the greater the degree of supervision that will be required. Trips to the home of a family member or to a familiar holiday destination are tolerated best. There is much to be said for staying in self-catering accommodation, minimizing the potential for embarrassment with other holiday makers. Often the travel is more disorienting than the final holiday; long coach and air journeys are especially difficult. A particular difficulty for couples can be using public toilets; a companion of the same sex who can accompany the person with dementia is a great help.

Many people prefer to take holidays in groups that can provide support to enable the primary caregiver to take some rest. Eventually a stage is usually reached where the person with dementia ceases to go on disorientating holidays and spends the time in respite care whilst their carer takes a break.

Some organizations (e.g. Vitalise in the UK) specialize in holidays for people with dementia and their carers at accessible holiday centres, but they are very popular and need to be booked well in advance. There is dual benefit as the carers can network with each other in addition to gaining an enjoyable break for all involved.

Summary

1. People with dementia need detailed baseline assessment and regular follow-up and monitoring of their progress. Community teams can help maintain people with dementia in their own homes and support informal carers.
2. Other community provisions such as day care and domiciliary care may also be valuable. Resources should be reviewed to check that they remain effective.
3. There are indicators that show when abuse of people with dementia may be occurring and there should be policies for dealing with this.
4. Driving is a worry for people with dementia and their families. Where there is doubt about fitness to drive, specialist assessment is valuable.

Treatment

Cognitive symptoms

The effectiveness of drugs to improve cognitive symptoms has been questioned, but worthwhile improvements can often be obtained by the appropriate prescription of anti-dementia drugs. Psychological treatments are comparably effective, although not always widely available. It is helpful to distinguish between treatments that seek to address the cognitive deterioration that dementia brings and those that target its psychological and behavioural consequences.

Drug treatments for cognitive symptoms

Before starting anti-dementia drugs it is worth checking that no medications are being taken that may be exacerbating cognitive impairment.

Many drugs have antimuscarinic properties. These include:
- Tricyclic antidepressants: especially amitriptyline and dosulepin.
- Antimuscarinic agents for Parkinsonism: procyclidine, orphenadrine, and trihexyphenidyl.
- Bowel antispasmodics: dicycloverine and propantheline.
- Bladder antispasmodics: tolterodine, oxybutynin, and trospium. These tend not to cross the blood-brain barrier and are less likely to cause problems, but they can cause confusion.

Other drugs that may cause a dementia-like syndrome include:
- Antiepileptic: especially older long-acting drugs such as phenytoin and phenobarbital.
- Lithium.
- Opiates.

Acetylcholinesterase inhibitors

Who benefits?

Acetylcholinesterase inhibitors (AChEI) are effective in improving cognition and slowing decline in cognition and skills required for ADLs in Alzheimer's disease and vascular dementia (📖 Box 6.1). However, the effects are relatively small (in the order of 1–4 MMSE points) and vary from person to person, some being apparent 'non-responders'. Changes in function and behaviour are more difficult to measure. Benefits are definite, but controversy surrounds whether they are generally large enough to really impact on individuals' lives. Dramatic benefits are most likely in dementia with Lewy bodies. There is also evidence that rivastigmine is effective in Parkinson's disease dementia.
- In mild cognitive impairment there is little evidence that AChEI is effective in improving cognitive function or delaying progression to dementia, but they may still cause adverse effects.
- Current guidance from the National Institute of Clinical Excellence (NICE) in the UK recommends AChEI may be used in Alzheimer's disease when the MMSE score is 10–20/30 (📖 Box 6.2).
- Assessment by an OT is helpful where it appears that the MMSE score does not reflect the degree of impairment caused by the dementia. If this is not possible, the Bristol ADL scale may be of use (📖 Chapter 13 p. 330).

Box 6.1 Implications for practice

In clinical trials, treatment with a cholinesterase inhibitor produced an improvement of 2.7 points (95% CI 2.3–3.0) on the 70 point ADAS-Cog scale. There were also improvements in global ratings made by clinicians blind to other measures. There were also benefits on ADL and behaviour rating scales. None of the effects of treatment was great. There were no significant differences between donepezil, galantamine, or rivastigmine in efficacy, but in one trial there were fewer adverse events reported for donepezil than galantamine.

Birks, J. Cholinesterase inhibitors for Alzheimer's disease. *Cochrane Database of Systematic Reviews* 2006; Issue 1. Art. No.: CD005593. DOI: 10.1002/14651858.CD005593.

Box 6.2 NICE guidance (http//:www.nice.org.uk)

The three acetylcholinesterase inhibitors donepezil, galantamine, and rivastigmine are recommended as options in the management of people with Alzheimer's disease of moderate severity only (in general those with a Mini-Mental State Examination (MMSE) score of between 10 and 20 points), and under the following conditions.

- Only specialists in the care of people with dementia (that is, psychiatrists including those specializing in learning disability, neurologists, and physicians specializing in the care of the elderly) should initiate treatment. Carers' views on the patient's condition at baseline should be sought.
- Patients who continue on the drug should be reviewed every 6 months by MMSE score and global, functional, and behavioural assessment. Carers' views on the patient's condition at follow-up should be sought. The drug should only be continued while the patient's MMSE score remains at or above 10 points and their global, functional, and behavioural condition remains at a level where the drug is considered to be having a worthwhile effect. Any review involving MMSE assessment should be undertaken by an appropriate specialist team, unless there are locally agreed protocols for shared care.
- The MMSE should not be relied upon in isolation in circumstances such as sensory or learning disabilities or communication difficulties.

NICE TA 111, Donepezil, galantamine, rivastigmine (review) and memantine for the treatment of Alzheimer's, pp 4–5.

November 2006, amended September 2007.

Starting treatment

Before starting on medication a full physical and psychiatric review should be carried out.

Families are often more enthusiastic than people with dementia about the possible benefits of treatment, and it is important to ensure, wherever possible, that the person who is going to take the medication is in agreement with this line of therapy.

In practice these medications rarely cause serious adverse effects but they need to be used with caution in people with:

- Obstructive airway disease.
- Peptic ulcer.
- Cardiac conduction disorders.

AChEI enhance parasympathetic activity, which may cause:

- Slowing of the heart rate.
- Increased GI tract motility.
- Lowering of intra-ocular pressure.
- Constriction of the airways.
- People with DLB are prone to carotid sinus hypersensitivity and other autonomic abnormalities. Use with care where there is a history of falls.

The commonest side effects are on the GI tract:

- Anorexia.
- Nausea.
- Vomiting.
- Diarrhoea.

These are rarely severe; if nausea and vomiting are a problem, co-prescribing domperidone for a short period at times when the dosage of AChEI is increased is usually sufficient to overcome any difficulties.

- Rivastigmine is the most and donepezil the least likely to produce adverse effects.
- Donepezil and galantamine tablets may be given once daily; galantamine liquid and rivastigmine liquid and tablets need twice daily administration. Donepezil is only available in tablet form. Rivastigmine can also be used in the form of adhesive patches applied once daily, which may cause fewer GI side effects.
- The patient information leaflet for donepezil recommends taking the dose at bedtime, but this is not always good advice. Taking the medication at night is more likely to cause nightmares.
- Gastro-intestinal side effects are less likely if the medication is taken after a meal.
- It is usually most convenient for patients to take their medication after breakfast so long as they have a reasonable meal at this time.
- Start at the lowest dosage (donepezil 5 mg od, galantamine MR 8 mg od, rivastigmine 1.5 mg bd) and review after 4 weeks.

Monitoring

Benefit is usually interpreted as there being improvement, or at least no decline, in MMSE score, but carers are usually sensitive to changes in people with dementia and may observe increased levels of awareness and motivation or a decrease in repetitive speech or behaviour. There may be improvement in mood or a reduction in hallucinations, delusions, or agitation. Clock drawing tests and other measures of visuo-spatial functioning are more sensitive to improvements than the MMSE (📖 Fig. 13.1–4).

- If there is no deterioration in MMSE score and there are beneficial effects, continue on the current dose. Review after 3 months and then at 6-monthly intervals.
- If there is no benefit but there are no adverse effects, continue to increase the dose at 4-weekly intervals until the maximum dose is reached.
- If there is no benefit after treatment for 2 months at full dosage:
  - donepezil 10 mg od
  - galantamine MR 24 mg od
  - rivastigmine 6 mg bd,

then no response is likely and the medication should be stopped.

- Occasionally stopping abruptly does make matters worse; this usually means that the medication was in fact producing some benefit and should be restarted.
- If there has been a period of more than a week off medication, it is necessary to restart at the lowest dose and titrate the dose upwards again to prevent adverse effects.
- NICE recommend that cognition, behaviour, and ADL skills are regularly assessed in patients receiving AChEI, although it is not clear how continued monitoring of these aspects of dementia is helpful in clinical practice once an initial positive response to an AChEI has been identified.
- More important is the opportunity for regular contact between the specialist dementia team, the patient, and the carers. This ensures that, in addition to pharmacological treatment:
  - The best possible social and psychological care is being provided.
  - There is an opportunity for continuing education and guidance for people with dementia and their carers about likely developments in the course of the disorder. (It is not usually good practice to give a gloomy prognosis at the start of dementia, but if there are signs of rapid deterioration, all those involved need to be alerted.)
  - Appropriate administrative and legal reviews can be undertaken—
    -should driving be allowed to continue?
    -is there a need to make provision for future incapacity?

Changing treatment

There is not much difference between available medications in terms of effectiveness, but prolonged treatment with an AChEI may result in increased activity of butyrylcholinesterase and in theory using a drug that also inhibits this enzyme ought to be helpful. Rivastigmine has this property and may be worth trying if response to donepezil or galantamine is decreasing, but there is not much evidence for this.

When the level of benefit from AChEI is diminishing there may be benefit in adding memantine (see below). This is not approved by NICE.

Stopping treatment

Relatively little research has been done on the effects of AChEI in more advanced disease. The guidance that they should be stopped when the MMSE score falls below 10/30 is not based on any rigorous evidence.

There is a serious ethical dilemma in stopping medication that may be producing some benefit, merely because some arbitrary threshold is crossed. This is especially the case if a person with dementia is being well supported in their home environment. There is always the risk that withdrawing treatment may precipitate a crisis resulting in admission to institutional care. Once the person has left home it may be impossible to re-establish previous arrangements.

All AChEI have a tendency to increase arousal. Whilst this is helpful in patients who display apathy, it may make pacing, wandering, and aggressive behaviour more difficult to cope with, even when there is a beneficial effect on cognition. It is generally preferable to stop the AChEI if it does exacerbate difficult behaviour.

Donepezil has a particularly long duration of action; it may take a month or more for the effect of stopping treatment to become apparent. There may be some benefit from re-starting therapy if the clinical state of the person with dementia deteriorates rapidly, but there is nearly always significant loss of function as a result of the interruption of medication.

AChEI in vascular dementia

Many people with dementia have some signs of both Alzheimer's disease and vascular dementia. Clinical trials have shown some benefit from using AChEI in vascular dementia but this seems to be mostly in people who have a degree of gradual deterioration in between clear-cut strokes.

They do not seem to be helpful in 'pure' vascular dementia, but the presence of incidental vascular lesions on a brain scan does not preclude a response to AChEI in a person with a clinical history suggestive of Alzheimer's disease.

Memantine

Memantine is a reversible antagonist at n-methyl-d-aspartate (NMDA) receptors. It was originally assessed as a drug that might limit brain damage and disease progression if given to patients at an early stage of the disease, but it seems to be of little benefit in these circumstances.

There is evidence that it slows the rate of functional decline in advanced Alzheimer's disease. It may also be of value in the treatment of disturbed behaviour. Research to determine the value of memantine in advanced dementia, and whether there may be benefit in prescribing it alongside an AChEI, is in progress.

It has few serious side effects.

Ginkgo biloba

This is not a licensed product but it is widely available from health food stores and pharmacies. It is an extract of leaves of the maidenhair tree; these extracts are not standardized and may vary in potency and purity. There are some studies showing minor benefits from using Ginkgo extracts in dementia; the better-designed studies have less impressive results. No serious adverse effects have been described in patients receiving Ginkgo, but there is a potential for interaction with other medicines, particularly warfarin and aspirin.

Psychological treatments

A model of memory

The biological basis of memory and how it is affected by dementia is not understood. However, psychological research enables us to conceptualize processes of remembering, which can be used to assist people with memory difficulties. For a fuller account of this model a non-technical introduction can be found in *Your Memory—A user's guide* by Alan Baddeley (4th edition 2004), Carlton Books, London.

All memory initially derives from sensations (📖 Figure 6.1):
- Hearing.
- Seeing.
- Feeling.

Most psychological research on memory has been done using verbal material, either read or heard. (It is possible to remember more information if it is listened to, rather than read.) However, tastes and smells are also remembered, as are pictures and non-verbal sounds.

Information from the senses is held in the short-term memory, which acts as a working area for processing data.

Some facts and events are transferred from short-term memory to the long-term memory for future reference. Information from the long-term memory store has to be retrieved through the working store if it is to be used. To psychologists, long-term memory refers to any information that is retained for more than a few seconds. Memory tested after 1–2 minutes appears to be similar to memory tested days or months later.

Information may reach long-term memory as a result of conscious remembering (explicit memory) or simply get picked up as a habit (implicit memory). Explicit memory can be divided into 'semantic' memory (for general knowledge), and 'episodic' memory (for events, or other knowledge that is specifically learned) (📖 Box 6.3).

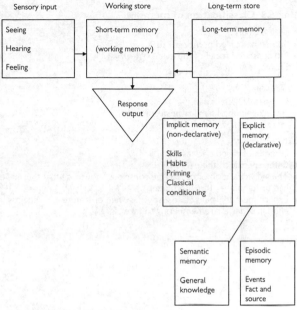

Fig. 6.1 A model of the memory system.

Box 6.3 Classification of memory

Implicit memory
- Sometimes called non-declarative.
- No conscious recall of the event of learning.
- Examples include:
  - reading
  - writing
  - basic ADLs
  - recognition of familiar environments
  - relationships.

Explicit memory
- Sometimes called declarative.
- Often specific to the person.
- The individual is able to describe conscious knowledge that they have had to remember the information.
- Explicit memory is linked to a specific event or feature and requires *effort* in order for remembering to take place.

Psychological approaches

Psychological approaches cannot reverse dementia and may not slow the underlying cognitive decline. Moreover, anything based on explicit new learning is likely to fail. 'Courses' of therapy are less likely to be effective than something that is embedded in everyday life and activity. Psychological approaches can be enabling—helping people with dementia improve performance, avoid complications (depression or anger), and reconnect with social experiences (for example by choosing activities, or groups of people with similar problems, where the individual can take part on a more equal footing).

Of many approaches that have been tried over the years, largely empirically and inadequately evaluated, three stand out as most effective: errorless learning, external memory aids, and cognitive stimulation therapy.

Cognitive rehabilitation and errorless learning

The development of person-centred approaches in dementia has led to a move away from purely disease-focused models and an increased awareness of the individual as they attempt to cope with the challenges of the disease by utilizing their remaining strengths.

Cognitive rehabilitation in dementia aims to enhance the quality of an individual's life rather than aspire to restore pre-morbid levels of cognitive functioning.

People with dementia rarely lose their memories completely and strategies explore the use of compensatory mechanisms that exploit existing cognitive systems or modify the individual's environment. Much of this area of research was originally conducted with people with head injuries or strokes and later adapted to dementia. The problems in acquiring new explicit memories and skills and the progressive nature of most dementias make this a particularly challenging area to demonstrate tangible benefits either clinically or in financial terms.

One approach that shows promise is 'errorless learning' (Box 6.4). This technique is particularly helpful for learning names of new social acquaintances or familiarizing oneself with new household appliances. Errorless learning aims to reduce or eliminate the number of incorrect or inappropriate responses that an individual makes during training. The rationale for this approach is that it reduces the processing load on an already impaired cognitive system. Individuals do not have to monitor and correct their own mistakes as errors are avoided during learning. In addition, the individual only experiences success during the training.

Box 6.4 Errorless learning

Learning how to use a cordless phone—for a person with impaired mobility and early dementia:

- Break down the task into easily managed elements.
- Start with the LAST—ending the call.
- Rehearse this until it becomes familiar.
- Move back to the previous element of the sequence.
- Rehearse again until the skill is acquired.
- Continue practising each item in turn until it becomes familiar, never going on until the current skill is thoroughly learned.

Using this technique the person with dementia will not experience the let down of failure but only the reward of success.

By learning the task in reverse ('reverse chaining') the part that is most difficult to remember—the last in the sequence—is the most practised.

External memory aids

External memory aids and strategies can be helpful. These are tools used to augment or substitute for memory. These range from the everyday (diaries, calendars, notice boards) to the more technologically advanced (palm top computers, pagers). Increasingly there is likely to be a cross-over in terminology with assistive technology. Interventions may include door alarms and medication boxes that prompt compliance with prescribed medication. Technically these could be seen as memory aids and they are certainly intended to maintain as much independence and autonomy as possible for the individual.

Cognitive stimulation therapy (CST)

There is considerable evidence for the effectiveness of CST, more so than other non-pharmacological interventions. It is derived from reality orientation approaches (RO), which prospered in the 1960s and 1970s. These techniques aimed to improve orientation by using a physical environment and conversation rich in cues for the person with dementia. However, many people with dementia did not enjoy being reminded how out of touch they were with the contemporary world. CST is more congenial to many people with dementia, with an emphasis on positive life experiences and person-centred care. Much of the demonstrable benefit of CST is in mood and morale, rather than cognition.

CST consists of structured group work organized around a number of consistent features (group song, orientation board, warm-up activity). It was initially designed as 14 'themed' sessions:

- Physical games.
- Sound.
- Childhood.
- Food.
- Current affairs.
- Faces/scenes.
- Word association.
- Being creative.

- Categorizing objects.
- Orientation.
- Using money.
- Number games.
- Word games.
- Team quizzes.

The programme is designed to be run over a 7-week period, but—unless resources dictate—there seems to be little rationale for its time-limited nature. It is suitable for people with mild to moderate dementia, combining an emphasis on socialization and enjoyment with activities designed to stimulate cognition.

In reality many activities that people with dementia find pleasurable, such as doing puzzles and crosswords, social conversation, and reminiscing, are actually forms of cognitive stimulation.

The evidence

Published studies have tended to have small sample sizes (often single case designs) and many have lacked control groups. At this time few studies have explicitly linked the use of learning strategies with helping individuals consistently use memory aids, and even fewer have done this within a group format.

Whilst the majority of interventions in this area have targeted individuals, some investigators have explored the use of group formats and shown positive benefits both from the content of the sessions and the experience of meeting others with similar difficulties.

It is possible to differentiate between interventions that have targeted explicit and implicit memory systems. The majority of interventions have focused on explicit memory and have achieved only modest success.

Compliance has been a problem due to memory difficulties.

Conclusions

The most helpful cognitive rehabilitation techniques appear to be implicit learning and external memory aids, and there may be benefits to providing cognitive rehabilitation in a group.

Behavioural and psychological symptoms in dementia (BPSD)

Behavioural problems, often resulting from psychological and emotional disturbance, are common in dementia—whatever the underlying pathology. They most frequently become an issue in the middle stages of the disease, as the ability to make sense of experience is diminished and decision-making by the person with dementia becomes more difficult. However, disturbed behaviour may occur much earlier (□ Box 6.5).

In addition to causing serious distress to people with dementia themselves, they are particularly difficult and upsetting for carers. They are the commonest reasons for people with dementia being admitted to hospitals or care homes. These difficulties are sometimes brought together under the term 'behavioural and psychological symptoms of dementia' (BPSD). This does not represent a single syndrome but BPSD rating scales (□ Chapter 13 p. 330) are useful checklists to use when seeing people with dementia and their carers.

Appropriate care (□ Chapter 4 p. 94–101) should always be the first approach to managing behaviour difficulties. There is little experimental evidence to support the use of any drug (or non-drug) treatment for BPSD, despite the size and severity of the problem, the frequency with which drugs are used, and the potential for side effects.

Common symptoms

- Agitation:
  - restlessness
  - inappropriate activity
  - following carer
  - wandering.
- Anxiety:
  - repeated questioning
  - fear of being left alone
  - phobias
  - fears in relation to personal care—washing, undressing etc.
- Apathy.
- Depression:
  - emotional lability
  - sustained low mood.
- Sleep disturbance:
  - daytime drowsiness
  - night-time wakefulness
  - day-night reversal.
  (Dramatic changes in sleep when person with dementia suddenly falls asleep and can't be roused or falls from a chair suggest DLB.)
- Aggression:
  - verbal aggression
  - physical aggression
  - aggression at times of personal care
  - spontaneous aggression
  - aggression in response to psychotic symptoms.

- Delusions/false beliefs:
  - 'understandable delusions'
    - beliefs of being abandoned
    - things are being stolen
    - people are coming to the house
    - this is not my home
    - I am being held here against my will
    - people are not who they say they are
    - 'mirror sign'—believing that reflections of faces in a mirror are other people
    - people on TV are real
  - 'psychotic delusions'
  - depressive delusions.
- Hallucinations:
  - related to sensory deprivation—misinterpreting ambiguous shapes e.g. patterns on carpets or curtains
  - strangers in the home
  - animals
  - hypnagogic hallucinations—occurring at times of dropping off to sleep and wakening.

Box 6.5 Epidemiology of behavioural and psychological problems

83% of people with dementia have symptoms at some point in their illness.

Table 6.1 Symptoms of dementia

Symptom	Percentage
Delusions	60%
Mood disturbance	40%
Anxiety	35%
Verbal outbursts	33%
Hallucinations	20%
Physical aggression	13%

64% of nursing home residents have significant behaviour problems.

International Psychogeriatric Association BPSD Task Force Report, 1996

Assessment

The commonest mistake is to institute drug treatment for BPSD, often under pressure from relatives or care home or hospital staff, out of a sense of desperation. The situation is 'intolerable' and 'something must be done'. Sometimes there is nothing that can be done, and management may entail helping others tolerate, or cope with, the behaviour.

On being presented with complaints of 'confused behaviour' or any other vague description, first of all ask 'What exactly do you mean?'
• Describe in detail what the behaviour is and when it happens.
• Does it vary throughout the day?
• Does anything precipitate it or bring it on?
• What happens afterwards?

Then you have a chance of understanding what is happening:
• Is it pain?
• Or fear?
• Need for the toilet?
• Does it occur during personal care tasks?
• When relatives leave?
• Is another patient or resident provoking?
• Is it in the evening (sundowning) or at night?
• Or more variable than that?
• Is difficult behaviour the prompt for special attention and activity?

Also make sure you know what diagnosis you are dealing with. Psychotic features, especially with variation in alertness or attention, suggest delirium or DLB. In both of these cases antipsychotic medication should be avoided.

Psychological treatments for BPSD

Appropriate communication and management

Whilst there is little research evidence that formal behavioural approaches have an impact on these difficulties, units with expertise in the management of people with dementia (be they hospital wards or care homes) do achieve less behavioural disturbance—with less use of drugs—than those that do not have such expertise, suggesting that some aspects of approach and communication can have an impact. These measures are an extension of the care approaches advocated in Chapter 4.

Insensitive communication and approaches can certainly make behaviour problems and psychological symptoms worse. Where the difficulties have been brought on by imperfect management, skilled handling and appropriate support can often alleviate them.

Behavioural management should centre on the assessment. If there is pain or a toileting issue, for example, then address these. The general rule is to avoid confrontation. Anger, threats, shouting, punishment, and reasoning never work. The key skills are anticipation and distraction.

Physical restraint as a means of behavioural control is generally thought unacceptable in the UK, other than in an emergency situation (when someone is at immediate risk of injuring themselves or someone else).

Meeting the needs of people with dementia for occupation and mental stimulation will reduce the overall incidence of disturbed behaviour, as will the availability of access to a quiet and relaxing environment.

Person-centred care (PCC)

This approach received acclaim as a result of the work of the late Tom Kitwood.

It describes an attempt to enhance carer awareness of the subjective world of people with dementia, in order to better understand their presentations (the 'phenomenological approach').

PCC does not exclude a biological basis for the cognitive impairment experienced by people with dementia, but it focuses on attempts to understand how such impairment may be presenting an individual with additional challenges and to provide an explanation for their behaviour (🕮 Box 6.6).

Box 6.6 PCC in practice

An individual may be disoriented in time and place but have intact recall. This essentially gives them a frame of reference that is 30 years in the past. It then becomes easier to understand why they are asking after a deceased partner and it is also not surprising that well-intentioned attempts to re-orientate them by reminding them about the bereavement are not welcome and only elicit anger and confusion.

Simply reassuring them that a deceased partner is merely absent may meet with more success. It may be possible to facilitate this by being 'economical with the truth' without 'lying' to an individual. It may also be helpful to ask the person about the underlying emotional content of their question (for example fear resulting from a degree of disorientation), which may help resolve the issue without addressing the superficial content of the question.

The application of PCC can raise difficult ethical dilemmas. Skilled individuals may be able to explore the meaning of the distress without effectively lying to the individual. However, other people may find themselves placating the individual with a well meant untruth such as 'Your wife/husband will be here later,' hoping that this white lie will not be remembered.

A central feature of PCC is that individuals with dementia are easily and often unintentionally denied their 'personhood' or value as an individual. Good care strives to maintain their sense of being in control of their actions and lives (*autonomy* and *agency*) as much as is realistically possible. Many psychological approaches to BPSD are grounded in PCC as a philosophy.

Maintaining a person-centred ethos in individual practice or In a care setting can be difficult for the carer. The principle is deceptively simple to grasp but very difficult to apply consistently. Good training, supervision, and reflection are paramount in supporting this approach.

Behavioural management

Any behavioural intervention or management programme should be based on a sound assessment, without which attempts to intervene can easily be experienced as traumatic and effectively become punishment.

Assessment of the individual's physical health should always be undertaken. Potentially treatable problems such as pain, constipation, and urinary tract infections should be excluded. People with dementia may experience delirium from infections or the side effects of medication. They may also be unable to communicate the presence of pain in ways other than through their behaviour.

In moderate to severe dementia, behavioural assessment may have to be largely based on observation, as a result of impairment of abstract thought, insight, and communication. However, levels of impairment should not be assumed and it is always advisable to attempt direct communication in the first instance.

Observational data can be structured and gathered in numerous ways. A commonly used structure is:
- A—antecedent.
- B—behaviour.
- C—consequence.

The observer can choose to record everything in a given period, or the most significant event or a targeted behaviour can be assessed for its frequency and intensity. Studying antecedents (A) may indicate potential causes that prompt the unwanted behaviour, whereas consequences (C) may reveal how such behaviour is being encouraged.

It is also possible to ask other people to gather data, although if they lack experience and have competing demands on their time they may be less effective than a trained observer.

Results must be analysed both on their own merits and in the context of the person's history.

Box 6.3

A residential home resident who repeatedly enters other residents' rooms and strips the beds may be difficult to understand without the context of a past history of work as a nurse or carer.

Sometimes very disturbed behaviour can be understood if an individual has a history of trauma or combat stress.

Using the ABC structure it may be possible to understand the specific behaviour sufficiently to intervene at the antecedent level and so prevent it from occurring. Alternatively alterations could be made that avoid an undesired consequence. Allowing an individual access to an area where they feel safe or can 'cool off' may prevent conflict from occurring.

With any behavioural intervention it is always necessary to consider the possibility that a particular environment is no longer appropriate for an individual, no matter what level of intervention or support is put in place.

Specific psychological therapies

A number of studies have examined the benefits of offering recently diagnosed individuals specific psychological therapies such as cognitive behavioural therapy, supportive counselling, systemic interventions, or psychodynamic psychotherapy.

The majority of interventions have focused on the process of adjustment.

Common themes are:
- To enable the expression of feeling of loss.
- To support people in addressing grief and other emotional reactions to the reality of having dementia.

- To encourage the sharing of experiences.
- To develop coping strategies.

Although the evidence base is small, there is evidence that relatively short programmes of therapy in individual and group formats can lead to statistically significant reductions in both anxiety and depression.

Drug treatments for BPSD

For many years the first line treatment for any behaviour disturbance or psychological symptom in a person with dementia was the prescription of medication. This was a misguided approach. Appropriate care (📖 Chapter 4) should always be the first approach to managing behaviour difficulties.

25–50% of nursing home residents with dementia are receiving antipsychotic medication. In the United States, federal regulations have restricted the use of these medicines in nursing homes since 1987; it appears that residents have benefited as a result.

Recently there have been concerns that antipsychotic agents cause an increase in deaths—particularly from stroke disease—and more rapid progression of dementia.

In the last 20 years, research to clarify the place of medication in the treatment of BPSD has been undertaken. This has confirmed that medication is of little value for many aspects of BPSD but may cause significant adverse effects. Much of this research has never been published.

Antidepressants

There has not been much research on the use of antidepressant medication in dementia.

Tricyclic drugs (amitriptyline and imipramine) are potently antimuscarinic and are likely to worsen cognitive impairment.

Paroxetine and fluoxetine are also poorly tolerated by people with dementia.

Trazodone and citalopram have been the most widely studied, and neither seems to cause serious problems. These drugs should be considered first if medication is needed for agitation, anxiety, or depression for a person with dementia.

- Trazodone:
  - generally well-tolerated with few adverse effects
  - may cause drowsiness or unsteadiness
  - if this is a problem give as a bedtime dose
  - helpful for anxiety and depressive symptoms
  - starting dose: 50 mg od or bd
  - increase by 50 mg per week up to maximum of 300 mg daily.
- Citalopram:
  - more potent antidepressant
  - especially useful for emotionalism in vascular dementia
  - may cause nausea, vomiting, and diarrhoea
  - not sedating
  - start at 10 mg od after food
  - increase by 10 mg every 1–2 weeks if necessary to maximum of 30 mg.

Sertraline is very similar (50 mg sertraline is equivalent to 10 mg citalopram). If one doesn't work there is no point in changing to the other.

Pathological emotionalism is often limited in time and medication can frequently be stopped after 2–3 months.

Agitated depression may respond better to trazodone but sertraline and citalopram are more effective for retardation. If neither trazodone nor citalopram work, mirtazapine (15–30 mg od) is worth trying, particularly for severe agitation or sleep disturbance, but it sometimes makes confusion worse.

Antipsychotics

These drugs have been widely used, particularly in care homes, for the treatment of a wide variety of symptoms. More prescriptions are issued for antipsychotics for treating dementia than for treating psychosis. Their use has frequently been criticized and there is evidence indicating that they may cause accelerated cognitive decline, strokes, and death.

A distinction is sometimes drawn between 'typical' (older and cheaper) and 'atypical' (newer and more expensive) antipsychotic drugs. It is claimed that the newer drugs have fewer Parkinsonian adverse effects. Such differences in side effects are small, only clozapine having a qualitatively different side effect profile, but it would practically never be justified to use this drug in people with dementia.

There is little evidence to suggest that they are of value in treating agitation, anxiety, or psychosis.

There is good evidence from controlled trials of risperidone and to a lesser extent olanzapine and haloperidol that they are effective in the treatment of aggression and aggressive agitation.

The same trials have shown that there is an increase in strokes and deaths in patients treated with active medication compared with placebo. Aripiprazole has been found to have the same adverse effects.

Management of aggression with antipsychotic medication is in our opinion justified where it is the least restrictive option when the safety and well-being of a person with dementia, their carers, or others who live with them, is put at risk.

Choice of drugs

- Haloperidol:
  - most likely to cause Parkinsonism
  - may cause less cardiovascular and metabolic effects
  - has been widely used in people with physical illness with little evidence of unexpected adverse effects
  - can be given in tablets, liquid, IM, or IV
  - liquid haloperidol is colourless, tasteless, and odourless (☐ covert medication p. 168)
  - initial dose 0.5–1 mg bd.
- Quetiapine:
  - less Parkinsonism
  - may be less likely to cause strokes or death
  - less evidence of effectiveness
  - disliked by patients, has few beneficial effects
  - does accelerate the progression of dementia
  - initial dose 25–100 mg od.

- Risperidone:
  - best evidence for reducing aggression
  - possibly less effect in causing stokes and death than olanzapine or aripiprazole
  - possibly fewer metabolic effects than olanzapine or aripirazole
  - initial dose 0.5–1 mg bd.
- Olanzapine:
  - similar to risperidone
  - worth trying if risperidone is ineffective or not tolerated
  - can be given IM but not recommended as it interacts with benzodiazepines when given by this route
  - initial dose 2.5–5 mg od.
- Sulpiride:
  - not formally investigated but some experienced clinicians still find it a useful drug
  - starting dose 100–200 mg bd
  - amisulpride virtually identical pharmacologically but more expensive.

Other situations
- If these doses do not work, increase the dose slowly by 50% each week (i.e. haloperidol 0.5 mg bd may be increased to 0.5 mg tds) to see if the desired result can be obtained.
- Increasing doses too fast may cause akathisia (restlessness) and exacerbate the problem.
- If Parkinsonian side effects occur, don't routinely use antimuscarinic medication (procyclidine, trihexyphenidyl). This may make the confusion and agitation worse. Instead reduce the dose or try a different drug.
- After 1–2 months try reducing the drug dosage; stop it completely if possible.

It is not a good idea to withdraw medication shortly before patients are discharged from hospital; a change of environment often causes a worsening of behaviour. It is better practice to reassess the patient in the new surroundings and adjust dosage there.

The poor showing of antipsychotic medicines in studies of psychosis in dementia may be partly due to problems with trial design or inappropriate rating scales that were used in the research. A trial of risperidone, olanzapine, or haloperidol (doses as above) is reasonable in patients with troublesome psychotic symptoms, particularly paranoid delusions or auditory hallucinations.

Patients with dementia with Lewy bodies are especially sensitive to the adverse effects of antipsychotic medication. In such patients quetiapine is less prone to produce Parkinsonism. Try 25 mg od or bd to start (well below the licensed dose) and increase up to the point where side effects become distressing or an effect is seen. Some patients may tolerate other antipsychotics; as ever start at low doses and don't increase too fast. It is difficult to give firm guidelines but monitor side effects and mental state on a daily basis.

Cholinesterase inhibitors such as rivastigmine may be effective and cause less Parkinsonism when treating psychosis in DLB.

Rapid tranquillization

If aggression is posing a risk to others it may be necessary to start at a higher dose, or to consider covert medication (📖 p. 168).

In an emergency when there are real dangers to other patients or carers, and all other treatments have failed, try haloperidol 2.5–5 mg IM. If this doesn't work add lorazepam 0.5–1 mg (📖 Table 3.2 p. 61).

Hypnotics

If the problems are mainly occurring during the night, it may be possible to reduce disturbance by using sleeping medication (📖 Chapter 4 p. 90). The heavier sleep brought on by medication may prevent waking and exacerbate difficulties with incontinence, but some carers will find this an acceptable compromise. There is no reliable evidence to guide the practitioner in the choice of medication. Temazepam (10 mg) and 'Z' hypnotics (zopiclone, zolpidem, and zaleplon) may be effective.

Clomethiazole (192–384 mg at night), which has a short half-life and rapid of onset of action, was used widely in the past and is worth considering as it tends to cause less hangover than other hypnotics. Clomethiazole is also licensed for the treatment of daytime confusion in older people; it may be helpful in the short term but if given more than once a day tolerance and dependence rapidly develop.

Where hypnotics are the best way of controlling severe behaviour disturbance or carer stress, it is justified to continue their use beyond the normal period of up to 4 weeks.

A rational approach to treatment

Delusions

Some delusions are an understandable reaction to cognitive impairment, for example:

- I'm being kept a prisoner here.
- You're not my husband/wife.
- This isn't my house.
- Someone has stolen my spectacles.

Try to understand such symptoms from the person with dementia's point of view and adjust your approach to them in the light of this.

Indications for antipsychotic drug treatment

- More bizarre psychotic delusions or ideas.
- When psychological therapies are ineffective.
- Where physical aggression is provoked by the delusion.

Anxiety and depression

Indications for antidepressant medication

- Anxiety or depression that still causes distress after psychological approaches have been attempted.
- Pathological emotionalism (📖 Chapter 1 p. 8).
- Biological symptoms of depression (📖 Chapter 1 Box 1.5).

Verbal outbursts

- Using a person-centred approach should minimize these.
- Consider pathological emotionalism. This is common in people with a vascular element in their dementia and may respond to an antidepressant.

Hallucinations

- Often due to sensory deprivation:
  - are they wearing glasses?
  - are the glasses the correct prescription and clean?
  - is the lighting appropriate?
  - consider rearranging the seating arrangements so that the area around the patient is clearly illuminated
  - patterned carpets, curtains, and wallpaper may exacerbate the problem
  - do they have wax in their ears?
  - is their hearing aid working?
  - could it be the television or radio?
- Consider dementia with Lewy bodies (📖 next page).
- Is it delirium due to illness or medication?

Physical aggression

If this occurs despite appropriate psychological approaches, an antipsychotic will need to be considered. Unless there is a contra-indication, try low-dose risperidone first.

Treatment of psychological difficulties in DLB

Dementia with Lewy bodies (📖 Chapter 1 p. 10) is the most 'biological' of all the forms of dementia and getting medication right is crucial. The basic principles of drug treatment (📖 p. 160) still apply. Agitation and psychosis are often caused by medication prescribed for the motor effects of Parkinsonism (📖 Chapter 9, p. 260).

- Try to stop all drugs for Parkinson's disease.
- Don't use antimuscarinic antiparkinson's drugs (orphenadrine, procyclidine, trihexyphenidyl).
- If medication is required, levodopa combinations (co-beneldopa, co-careldopa) have the best therapeutic profile and are least likely to exacerbate psychological problems. Avoid dopamine agonists, MAO-B inhibitors (selegiline), and COMT inhibitors (entacapone).
- AChEI are less likely to cause problems than antipsychotics, but there are sometimes autonomic abnormalities in DLB and cardiovascular side effects need to be considered.
- Hallucinations in DLB may respond to AChEI. If there is real distress consider an antipsychotic; if DLB is a real possibility try quetiapine first.
- Depression in DLB may be due to biochemical disturbance rather than life events. Citalopram is a good choice of antidepressant.

Second line treatments

Memantine

Memantine is relatively ineffective in early disease but it does appear to slow decline in advanced dementia and may be of some value in treating BPSD. It causes few side effects.

Antiepileptics

A clinical trial of carbamazepine in patients with BPSD suggested that this drug might have some beneficial properties. However, it is very prone to cause excess sedation (and some metabolic effects, such as SIADH). The majority of patients in whom it is tried do not tolerate it. Other antiepileptics such as valproate have also been evaluated but the results of these studies have been disappointing. Where other treatment options have proved ineffective and behaviour disturbances continue to cause difficulties, a course of antiepileptic medication may be considered.

Start with sodium valproate 100–200 mg bd and increase up to 1 g daily. Once the correct dose has been established, use modified release tablets once daily to make the medication regime simpler. Withdraw slowly if it is ineffective (over 1–2 months) to avoid withdrawal fits.

Acetylcholinesterase inhibitors

Acetylcholinesterase inhibitors (AChEI) are somewhat stimulating in their effects and may be helpful if apathy is a problem; conversely they may make agitation and anxiety worse. However, a recent controlled trial showed no impact of AChEI on agitation in people with dementia. They may also be helpful for visual hallucinations and other symptoms of psychosis, particularly in people with DLB. People with DLB may be especially sensitive to cardiovascular adverse effects of AChEI.

Anxiolytics

The studies that have been carried out with these drugs have not shown much benefit, and they can cause increasing confusion, unsteadiness, and drowsiness. They may still have a place for symptomatic relief of severe agitation. Some authorities advocate the use of short-acting agents such as lorazepam and oxazepam and these can be helpful in the emergency situation, but in longer-term use they are likely to cause increasing agitation as their effect wears off after a few hours. For the few individuals who have long-term distress not adequately relieved by psychological measures or antidepressant medication, low doses of diazepam (2 mg od or bd) or chlordiazepoxide (5–15 mg daily) can be a great kindness.

Aromatherapy

Hand massage with oils containing aromatic fragrances has been shown to be of some value in the short-term reduction of agitation in people with dementia. No adverse effects have been reported and the research subjects seem to enjoy the experience.

Many other treatments have been tried for BPSD; none has shown any conspicuous signs of effectiveness.

Review

BPSD are generally limited in time and often remit after a few months. It is important to keep all medications under regular review to see if they are still worthwhile (at least monthly at home or in care homes and at least weekly in hospital).

Covert medication

What should you do for a person who refuses medication? Are there circumstances that justify you deceiving a patient into taking medication?

Giving medicine covertly, that is, disguised in food or drink, is widely practised. 70% of care homes admit to sometimes doing this. Several supervisory and professional bodies have considered this and there is general agreement about the circumstances when covert administration of medication is justified.

- The patient lacks capacity to make decisions on medical treatment (📖 Chapter 11 p. 285).
- The treatment is necessary.
- The treatment is in the patient's best interests (📖 Chapter 11 p. 288).
- Covert administration of medication is the best way to achieve the desired goal.

Before starting treatment there should be a multidisciplinary review and discussion with the patient's family and friends. Treatment should only be started if there is a consensus that covert treatment is the best way forward. It is important to include a pharmacist in this review to check that the proposed treatment can be given in this way.

There should be regular reviews to confirm that covert medication is still required. The Mental Welfare Commission for Scotland (http//:www.mwcscot.org.uk) has produced helpful checklists for use before starting treatment and for reviewing the practice. The precise legal details will vary in other countries, but the principles are the same.

Summary

1. Acetylcholinesterase inhibitors are effective in improving cognitive functioning in Alzheimer's disease, but the effects are not great. More improvement sometimes occurs in dementia with Lewy bodies.
2. Psychological approaches are also effective; any form of pleasurable stimulation is beneficial.
3. Behavioural and psychological difficulties are common and distressing for people with dementia and their carers. Behavioural and communication approaches are the first line in management.
4. Antipsychotic medication is often used, and may sometimes help, but often doesn't suppress symptoms without also causing unacceptable side effects. Use only in emergencies, or as a last resort, and review critically for effectiveness and side effects.

Summary

Care homes for people with dementia

Introduction

The purpose of this chapter is to assist readers in understanding issues surrounding admission of people with dementia into care homes and some of the problems that can arise there. The principles of care in Chapter 4 are also applicable in care homes.

About two thirds of all residents in care homes in the UK have dementia, about 370 000 people. Half of all people aged over 65 with dementia live in care homes. The prevalence of dementia in residents increases from about 55% among those aged 65–69 to about 65% in those aged 95 and over.

The annual cost of dementia in the UK is £17 billion, more than the combined cost of stroke, heart disease, and cancer. Much of this is spent on institutional care. The average annual cost for a person with dementia in a care home is over £31 000. The pressure to reduce costs has led to many staff being paid at around the national minimum wage. Homes are often staffed by workers from overseas with little understanding of English language and customs, which can limit the quality of relationships that they are able to develop with their clients. These staff may have more than one job in an attempt to achieve financial security. The market economy is not ideally suited to providing a service to vulnerable people. As one carer reported: 'The only homes that ever have vacancies are those you wouldn't want to put a dog in. The decent homes always have waiting lists that are years long.'

Staff in care homes are expected to maintain high professional standards, remain cheerful and vigilant, and to show high awareness of legislation on health and safety at work, non-discrimination, and the principles of person-centred care. It is essential that they show respect, courtesy, and dignity to people who may not be able to communicate with them, who may be immobile, incontinent, and who may subject them to psychological and physical abuse. Care staff are frequently portrayed in the media as being aggressive and unconcerned.

Abuse of residents in care homes (📖 Chapter 5 p. 128) occurs mostly at the hands of younger staff who get little satisfaction from their work, are stressed in their own lives, have conflict with their superiors, and have been subject to aggression from those for whom they care. These difficulties are frequently compounded by a lack of training in how to provide care, how to recognize early warning signs that there is a risk of aggression, and how to reduce these risks. One survey found that 85% of care home workers reported being psychologically abused by people in their care in the previous month; 60% had been the victims of physical abuse. On average a carer could expect to be assaulted 9.3 times each month and insulted 11.3 times. In another 200-bed nursing home, 8 days of observation revealed 182 acts of physical aggression against staff, resulting in 11 significant injuries.

Regulations controlling minimum standards of room dimensions and other aspects of the environment are easy to inspect and enforce but it is more difficult to capture the atmosphere and quality of personal relationships that really makes the difference for residents.

Despite all this there are homes that try hard to offer the best possible standards of care, that maintain a friendly and cheerful atmosphere and comfortable surroundings with well-motivated and committed staff who achieve good relationships with relatives and friends of the residents.

The move to long-term residential care

Most of us are desperate to carry on in our own homes and at best will only settle for institutional living reluctantly. The decision to look for long-term care for someone with dementia is laden with powerful emotions of loss and guilt. For a partner of many years it represents the end of a living arrangement that has lasted most of their adult lives. For them, and for those acting as the main carer of a parent with dementia, it can feel like the ultimate act of betrayal, however much they acknowledge rationally that they are 'doing the right thing'. These feelings should not be underestimated by home managers when they meet enquirers for the first time.

Such is the difficulty of making decisions about long-term care that many people will put off thinking about and discussing the issue until events force it upon them—such as a sudden turn for the worse in the person with dementia or their carer.

Decisions made in such haste are best avoided and it is important, therefore, that involved professionals provide a framework or forum for thinking about long-term care decisions well in advance of the anticipated time that residential care is needed.

Making the right decision

A move to a care home may be inevitable. But some people decide that they would rather not have the burden of domestic responsibility, or prefer the comfort and relative security of a care home (subject to this decision being financed, either by the individual themselves or by Social Services). Others are distressed by spending so much time alone and relish the prospect of company. Sometimes a couple with varying degrees of individual infirmity will decide to move to a care home together.

Some families hold an unduly rosy view of what life in a care home is like, but there is a very high prevalence of disability (Table 7.1). 27% of all care home residents are confused, immobile, and incontinent.

In many cases a decision to move is made in a crisis, or with a sense of desperation. There appears to be no other option. Health and social care services should ensure that as many options are made known and available as possible. This should include:

- A comprehensive multidisciplinary assessment.
- Identification of problems that can be cured or alleviated or may be amenable to rehabilitation.
- Assessment of the expectations, needs, and preferences of the person with dementia and their family.
- Exploration of the risks and benefits of possible courses of action.
- Consideration of how decisions can best be made.
- Support in decision-making.
- Provision of adequate support services to assist in remaining at home, even if only in the short term (perhaps a 'trial' period).
- Backup plans if the first choice doesn't work.

Table 7.1 Common problems in care homes

Problem	Percentage of residents with problem	
	Nursing homes	**Residential homes**
Impaired mobility	82%	60%
Incontinence	80%	50%
Mental disorder	80%	70%

Support networks

Many factors may influence the decision to move into residential care (📖 Box 7.1). As a general rule, the stronger the support network, the longer the person with dementia can remain at home (📖 Box 7.2). Household composition is the single most important determinant. The person with dementia who lives with a partner and/or other family members can obviously draw on more supervision and support than those who live alone.

Other important 'informal' sources of support include neighbours and friends who live locally; also wardens of sheltered housing who sometimes go well beyond their designated roles.

Carer strain

The demands placed upon carers are variable, particularly in relation to the person with dementia:

* Behaviour—Many people with dementia retain a strong sense of attachment to their own homes and feel secure there, but family members are frequently worn down by the emotional demands placed on them. They are likely to resent being induced to feel guilt every time a break is taken from caring or even being the victims of verbal and physical aggression.
* Cognitive deficits—The need to remain constantly alert in order to supervise someone who is no longer able to keep themselves safe causes stress to the point of exhaustion in carers. Carers vary greatly in what they find stressful, but regular disturbance of sleep, clearing up faecal incontinence, and being subject to violence are nearly always intolerable if they continue for any length of time. Not being recognized and not getting any response from the person for whom one is caring also wears down carers.
* Physical health—Physical health may also impact upon the tolerance of carers, especially if it affects mobility or continence.

Intensity of care needs

Ultimately the root cause of a move is usually that the need for care exceeds the available supply of help. Sometimes the person with dementia themselves will not share the view of others involved in the decision-making about the amount of care needed or the level of risk involved in their continuing to live at home.

Example 7.1

Mr G. had dementia and lived with his wife, with support from their daughter who lived nearby and herself had two children with learning disabilities. Mrs G. and her daughter met at regular 3-monthly intervals with Mr G.'s social worker and community psychiatric nurse. These meetings reviewed the current care package of home care, day care, and respite care, as well as providing an opportunity to think together about the longer term. Through these discussions Mrs G., who had significant health problems herself, was able to identify the potential extent and type of difficulties in caring for Mr G. that would be too much for her to cope with. She was able to agree with her daughter that these would serve as the 'threshold' beyond which they would start looking actively for long-term care.

Box 7.1 Personal factors for informal carers

- Work and other commitments.
- Health.
- Wishes and motivation.
- Quality of relationship.
- Willingness to accept help from others.
- Capacity to tolerate stress.
- Attitude towards risk.

Box 7.2 Other sources of support for carers

- Home care.
- Day care.
- Respite residential care.
- Befriending and sitting services.
- Family, friends, and neighbours.

Choosing a home

Finding a good care home: tips for families and friends

- Ask around—the local branch of the Alzheimer's Society or another voluntary body is often a good place to start.
- In the UK, inspection reports for all registered care homes can be downloaded from the Commission for Social Care Inspection (CSCI) website (www.csci.org.uk). The CSCI also produce checklists of questions to ask homes.
- Homes have to produce a statement of purpose and a service user guide—study these.
- Turn up at the home without asking for an appointment. Homes inevitably have a turnover of residents and are well used to enquirers and visitors. If nothing else, having seen two or three homes allows a more informed discussion of the issues and possibilities.
- Spend some time in the communal living areas to see what life is going to be like. Talk to the families who visit the home.
- If you see things that concern you in an otherwise good home, ask to see the manager to seek an explanation.
- Raise with management anything that concerns you about an inspection report.
- Atmosphere and the quality of interactions and relationships between residents and staff are better indicators of suitability than the quality of fixtures and fittings. It is unrealistic to expect a home that caters for people who may be aggressive or prone to wander to be as well maintained as one where all the residents are immobile.
- Think about current and future need: when considering the type of living arrangement that will best meet the needs of someone with dementia it is important to keep in mind the progressive nature of the condition.
- If available, short-term respite care can provide an opportunity to test the suitability of placements prior to decisions about long-term care being taken.
- Short-listing:
  - Is the home in the right place—will it be possible for visitors to call regularly?
  - Will it be possible to pay the bills of this home?
  - If you can't, will somebody else (e.g. local authority social services)?
  - Is this home going to continue to be suitable if the condition progresses?
  - What happens if the partner also requires a care home—but maybe not for dementia?
  - Consider waiting lists and available room types.

Residential respite care

If a move into a care home seems imminent, a planned short period of residential care can answer many questions.

However, it may destabilize a person who had been coping at home with domiciliary social care support to the point when at the end of their short stay they never manage at home again.

If the short stay goes well, it is worth reviewing the care plan, incorporating what has been learned.

It is important for the self-esteem of some carers to feel that they are the only people who can provide appropriate care for their family member. Their complaints about poor care in an institution may reflect this, but actual poor care is a more likely explanation.

In many places units that provide day care are attached to residential units; it causes much less disruption if residential respite can be provided in a familiar setting, with an opportunity for people who know the person from day care to also keep in touch whilst they are in on respite. Sadly, it is not always possible to arrange longer-term placement in the same unit if this becomes necessary.

Generic care home or specialized dementia unit?

There is no single right answer to this difficult question. It will depend on the particular abilities and problems of the person concerned, and what is available locally. In some countries (including the UK) there are special regulatory requirements for homes managing people with dementia.

- Specialist homes hopefully provide greater expertise, can deal with more severe problems, and in some situations achieve better outcomes. Community mental health teams may find it easier to work with better trained staff.
- Generic homes are likely to be more available locally, and will have a different mix of residents (but remember that most residents in most homes have some evidence of dementia). They may be less tolerant of difficult or disturbed behaviours than specialist homes.
- Dementia will inevitably progress and future needs will change. Physical frailty will also increase (📖 Chapter 9).
- Problem behaviours are likely to settle down eventually, but may become more severe in the early stages after moving to an institution.
- Families and people with early dementia will often feel easier with a home where other residents have relatively mild levels of impairment or disturbance. If people who are more seriously affected predominate in a home, this may cause the newcomer to retract within themselves, rather than make efforts to socialize with other residents.
- If a home has residents with mild levels of cognitive impairment and little disturbed behaviour, it may indicate a care regime where residents are kept stimulated and active, slowing the progression of the disorder.
- Alternatively, it may indicate a lower threshold of tolerance towards such problems.
- Most people are uncomfortable being in a setting where they are surrounded by people who are more cognitively impaired. However, some people with dementia may not object to being in an environment where the other residents are more disturbed than they are—this may

be their first experience of being the 'top dog' and they may enjoy the sensation (see Example 7.2).

Sometimes the staff at a home are prepared to be tolerant of unsettled behaviour in a newcomer, but the existing residents can make life difficult for the new arrival and exacerbate any minor problem until it becomes a justification for demanding removal. It is crucial to get the initial phase right; this may be a time when resorting to medication for a short time to minimize disruptive behaviour is justified.

Homes are often prepared to keep on a resident who creates more disturbance as their condition progresses, and sometimes specialized treatment (🕮 Chapter 6) may ease the problem. However, sometimes it is better to accept the inevitable and recognize that a move to new surroundings is better than trying to persevere with a failing placement.

Making a decision

Having arrived at a short-list it is important to involve the person with dementia in the final decision as much as is possible. It can be difficult for carers to gauge the view that the potential resident will take themselves.

Example 7.2

Mrs H. hesitated before taking her friend Mr D. to view Orchard Lodge, as she feared that the other residents were more cognitively impaired than he was and that he would find it too threatening to be amongst them. It became clear during the visit, however, that he was revelling in being amongst a group in which he felt he had some superior status—contrasting to the sense of humiliation that he seemed to recently experience amongst his 'cognitively intact' peers.

Entering a care home

Sooner or later?
- Early placement pros:
  - Skills (e.g. dressing, personal hygiene, toileting) that are retained on entry to the home are likely to be preserved. People with dementia living alone are likely to become more impaired, and once a skill is lost it is unlikely to be re-learned.
  - The person entering care can make a greater contribution to the choice of home.
- Early placement cons:
  - If the person really doesn't like the chosen home and they return to independent living, they are likely to be more resistant in the future if a placement becomes inescapable.
  - If they are dependent on Social Services to fund the placement, finance will not be available unless strict criteria are met.

Direct from home or via hospital?
Behaviour—rather than cognitive function or abilities with activities of daily living—is what usually precipitates a move into a care home. It is very difficult to arrange community services to support day-night reversal or wandering for someone living on their own.

The sudden emergence of these symptoms—even if they are due to a potentially reversible cause—may make continued independent living impossible. If a place in a suitable home is available and there are no health needs for diagnosis or treatment to make hospital essential, then moving straight to a care home is often best. Hospitals have to be able to deal with the most serious medical and psychiatric problems; although ward staff are often highly skilled and professional it is usually impossible to maintain a welcoming and supportive environment for a person with uncomplicated mild dementia on a hospital medical admission ward.

On the other hand, if the person's behaviour is very disturbed a brief period in hospital to identify and treat the underlying causes may permit an informed assessment of the best future care plan.

(In reality, after the brief assessment, the delay in implementing an agreed plan whilst the right home or the necessary community support becomes available can result in prolonged hospital admission with complications and further deterioration.)

Care home staff

New staff, new problems?

Care homes are only as good as the people who work there.

Nothing affects the atmosphere of a home as much as the person in charge. A good new head arriving may take months to turn around a failing home, but the arrival of a poor manager can quickly ruin the atmosphere of a previously good home.

Support from health and social care professionals may help to improve matters, but sometimes it may be necessary to consider moving residents if the new management can't offer them a reasonable life.

Supporting care home staff

Members of community health and social care teams have many skills that can be of great value to people in care homes. Some homes are eager to have guidance and education from members of a specialist team.

By offering regular input to care homes it is possible to enhance the ability of people with dementia to be looked after in a home of their choice, rather than being forced into the only home that is prepared to take them on.

Abuse of people with dementia

People with dementia are vulnerable, and abuse is regrettably common in hospitals and care homes. Many of the issues are the same as for abuse occurring at home (⌐ Chapter 5 p. 128).

- Many organizations have a role in preventing, detecting, and monitoring abuse. All prospective employees and volunteers need to be checked with the Criminal Records Bureau and under Protection of Vulnerable Adults procedures before they are taken on.
- Care workers who have harmed a vulnerable adult or placed a vulnerable adult at risk of harm (whether or not in the course of their employment) are banned from working in a care position with vulnerable adults.
- Anyone who employs a care worker is bound to report an employee who is guilty of misconduct that harmed or placed at risk a vulnerable adult.
- The Mental Capacity Act has introduced a new offence in England and Wales, of wilfully neglecting a person without capacity.

There are pressures on both professional and informal carers, and those who are employed to attend to a person who needs care need support and supervision themselves. It is clear that stress in paid carers predisposes to abuse, and supporting them can help mitigate the worst consequences. Education about the nature of dementia and how to communicate best with people with dementia can be of great benefit.

What to do about suspected abuse

If you become aware that a member of staff at a care home (or hospital) is abusing people for whom they should be caring, you should initially draw this matter to the attention of the responsible manager. If the registered person in charge of a care home fails to act upon this information they may be unsuitable to be running the home.

In the UK, local authorities are required to have policies in place to investigate and manage suspected cases of abuse. Social Services usually act as lead agency for these procedures (often referred to as 'Vulnerable Adults Policies'). In England and Wales an Independent Mental Capacity Advocate (⌐ Chapter 11) should be appointed to safeguard the victim's interests.

Commission for Social Care Inspection (CSCI)

This is the body responsible for inspecting and licensing care homes, private hospitals, and care agencies. Where it is reasonably believed that individuals have been guilty of abuse they can be prevented from working with vulnerable adults. The CSCI maintains a register of people who have been found to be unsuitable to work with children or vulnerable adults.

Summary

1. Care homes have to operate in difficult circumstances; it is not surprising that sometimes they cannot satisfy everyone.
2. Wherever possible families should take time and care to select the best available home and ensure that the move to this environment is achieved with the minimum of distress.
3. Where care falls below an acceptable standard it is everybody's duty to report this to the appropriate authority.

Dementia and delirium in hospitals

People with confusion in general hospitals

This chapter is mostly about people with dementia in acute and rehabilitation geriatric and medical units, but much of it is also relevant to psychiatric wards.

People with confusion may be admitted to general hospitals because:
- Confusion may be 'medical'—delirium, or suspected delirium, with or without prior dementia.
- There may be a medical (or surgical) problem in someone who has dementia, which requires investigation, treatment, or rehabilitation.
- Presentation may be non-specific and the relative contributions of medical, psychiatric, and social factors undetermined.
- Relatives, or GPs, may feel there is no alternative in a crisis, so people are admitted by default.
- Admission for elective surgery.
- People with dementia may also attend for tests, outpatient appointments, or day hospitals.

If you are going to be admitted to and then remain in hospital, it has to be for a purpose. Or at least, it is important that we understand what hospital has to offer. This is mainly because hospitals are no place to live a life, but also because there are hazards, and beds represent a scarce resource. Reasons for being in hospital include:
- Nursing care—skilled observation, feeding, washing, hygiene, basic mobility, protecting pressure areas, avoidance of other complications, and delivering medication, especially where care is required unpredictably or intensively 24 h a day.
- Access to diagnostic tests not available outside hospital.
- Access to medical and surgical treatments that are not available outside hospital.
- Delivery of rehabilitation, including rehabilitation nursing.
- Waiting—for tests, treatment, or for home or institutional care to be organized or available.
- Convenience of not requiring multiple trips to hospital for tests, therapy, or medical consultations.

The hospital environment

- What it provides:
  - relative safety
  - warmth
  - prompting
  - 24-h supervision
  - intensive physiological monitoring
  - access to doctors, nurses, therapists, and supervised drug therapy
  - explanation and discussion with relatives and carers
  - time for planning discharge and future care.
- What it may lack:
  - consistent availability of nurses and doctors familiar with (or sympathetic to) dementia, delirium, and behavioural approaches to management
  - occupation or diversion
  - quiet
  - close links with community services.
- Problems it can cause:
  - unfamiliarity causes disorientation, fear, agitation, or desire to leave
  - hospital-acquired infection
  - potential for deconditioning and unnecessary disability
  - disruption to or by other patients.

The key is to balance the risks and the benefits. Ask what hospital care can deliver that cannot be delivered equally well or more safely in another setting. That, of course, depends on what other settings are available locally. Possibilities include outpatient clinics, day hospitals, and intermediate and domiciliary care.

Some of these have problems in their own right. Domiciliary care can rarely provide round the clock supervision or rapid intervention in a medical crisis. Outpatient clinics, preceded by the disruption of having to get there and negotiate hospital car parking and sign-posting, can be equally strange and disorientating places, and a relatively brief appointment can give a poor impression of someone's usual abilities. A new outpatient appointment for someone with moderate or severe dementia will take at least an hour. Make each appointment count. Only arrange follow-up appointments where this is really necessary. Test results can often be communicated by letter or telephone, especially where there is no change in the management plan.

However, acute hospital care is not all bad. In particular, the 'front-end' of acute care provides a premium service, available 24 hours a day and 7 days a week, with the possibility of rapid diagnosis and emergency medical treatment.

Problems arise when inexperienced or inexpert staff:
- Fail to appreciate the need for mental state, functional, and social assessment.
- Fail to appreciate the nature or extent of problems (for example mistaking delirium for dementia, or being unsure how to investigate for a cause, or misdiagnosing depression).

- Fail to go through a comprehensive decision-making process before instituting (or withholding) invasive or aggressive treatments.
- Use, or over-use, of sedative or antidepressant drugs that cause side effects.
- Fail to recognize the need for rehabilitation or the length of the recovery time for delirium.
- Fail to approach rehabilitation appropriately, including being overly focused on difficulties with attention and retention ('carry over'), and apparent lack of consent.
- Fail to make adequate plans for follow-up or ongoing care.

The result is often a prolonged hospital stay, frustrated nurses, doctors and therapists, anxious or angry relatives, annoyed primary care staff, and a patient who is not given the opportunities or options for the future that they might have had.

Prevalence of mental health problems on medical wards

Like many things, this depends on how you define it and where you look. Table 8.1 gives some typical prevalence figures.

Table 8.1 Prevalence of mental health problems in different settings

	Delirium	Dementia	Depression
All people over 65	1%	5%	15%
All people over 80	2%	20%	20%
All hospitalized people over 65 (admission)	20%	25%	20%
Incident in hospital	10–20%	-	-
Acute general medical wards	10%	10%	10%
Acute geriatric medical wards	25%	50%	25%
Nursing home residents	10%	80%	50%

Effect of cognitive impairment on length of hospital stay

Both delirium and dementia increase length of stay. In one study of elderly acute medical emergency admissions, mean length of stay was increased from 8 to 14 days by the presence of delirium.

This is because of:
- Clinical complexity and diagnostic and therapeutic difficulty.
- The widespread need for functional assessment, rehabilitation, risk assessment, and discharge planning.
- Difficulties engaging in, and slowness of response to, rehabilitation therapy.
- The sometimes prolonged recovery time for delirium, required before sensible planning can take place.
- The need to negotiate with families and other carers.
- Liability to complications (falls, fractures).
- Delays in accessing diagnostic tests and opinions.
- Delays in accessing community support services or care home availability.

Risk of readmission is high, but this is not always a bad thing. A 'trial of discharge' is often necessary to ascertain if living at home is viable. Inevitably this will fail in a proportion of cases, providing information for ongoing planning.

Length of stay should be minimized by clear objective setting, timely comprehensive assessment of future care needs, and discharge planning. Specialist supported early discharge and intensive home support services and community mental health teams can help if available locally.

Ill health in older age

The classical medical approach to acute illness proceeds through several stages:

- Identify symptoms and signs to define a clinical syndrome (e.g. typical chest pain with associated symptoms in heart attack).
- Infer a pathology from the syndrome (e.g. myocardial infarction).
- Treat the pathology, and/or its complications (e.g. thrombolysis, drugs for heart failure or arrhythmias).
- Institute secondary prevention.
- Await functional restoration.

This approach is insufficient in the face of multiple pathologies and chronic or progressive diseases. The process of diagnosis remains important, and treating the treatable will often be helpful, but palliation, multidisciplinary management, information giving, counselling and negotiation of goals, restoration of function, and manipulation of the physical and social environment assume increased importance. A comprehensive initial assessment (📖 Chapter 2) is essential to avoid overlooking problems, causing difficulties and delays later on. Where an emergency team has conducted a preliminary evaluation, this needs to be completed later on.

Multiple pathology is a defining feature of ill health in old age. People with dementia often have other things wrong as well. Dementia, stroke, and hip fracture all increase exponentially with age. Arthritis, heart and lung problems, poor vision, deafness, and bladder problems are also common. Older people are also more prone to complications, and the adverse effects of treatments.

Pathologies may be acute (rapid onset, short-term, quickly leading to recovery or death), chronic (persisting, more or less stable), progressive (inexorably getting worse with time), or relapsing-remitting.

Older people are prone to rapid deterioration, often because of acute illness or injury. The severity of illness required to precipitate functional decline is less than in younger people. A minor viral infection may be sufficient to cause a crisis. The concept of 'frailty' includes both limitation in functional ability and vulnerability to deterioration.

One response to this is to concentrate on assessing functional ability, or disability. This includes physical capacity to perform various tasks or activities, but also embraces cognition, volition, and mood, and social and environmental aspects.

Diagnosis

Diagnosis is the process of explaining problems in pathological terms. Without it, logical further management—treatment, rehabilitation, prognostication—is difficult or impossible. See also Chapter 2.

Older people differ medically from their younger counterparts:
- Presentation is often non-specific or atypical. The classical non-specific presentations are confusion, immobility, falls, and incontinence, or an even less well specified 'inability to cope'.
- Diseases are multiple.
- Older people lose abilities fast—so diseases can present with their functional consequences.
- Older people are more prone to complications of diseases and their treatments.
- They are more dependent on the environment—someone with an adverse environment will present sooner, someone with a supportive environment often later, and presentation may be due to a change in the environment rather than the person.
- They need explicit rehabilitation.

This complicates diagnosis, which can be difficult, but is usually amenable to an approach thorough to the point of obsessiveness. Good care for older people is slow:
- If the patient is ill or unco-operative, at least try to take a history. Remember that fatigue and loss of attentiveness may limit the time you can spend, so be selective. Current symptoms are most likely to be reported accurately, the social situation and drug history will need confirmation regardless, and the family history is usually valueless. Assess the mental state at the same time.
- Take a proper third party history ('clerking the relatives') if the patient is unable or the story uncertain.
- Examine thoroughly, including mental state, nervous system, and joints. Be on the lookout for anything that might help (temperature, skin signs, the mouth). Dehydration cannot be assessed clinically in an older person. Chest examination is unreliable. If in doubt, order electrolyte and renal blood tests, and a chest X-ray. A lot can be determined without doing a formal examination (for example if the patient is not co-operative). Are there signs of distress, pain, or breathlessness? Visual fields, squint, facial weakness, swallow, limb movement, balance, and gait, can, with a little ingenuity, all be assessed with little more than observation.
- Comorbid physical conditions must be assessed fully. The aetiology of delirium is likely to be multi-factorial, the explanation for disabilities almost certainly so. You need all the help you can get; be on the lookout for as much that you can treat as possible (there will be plenty that you cannot).

Investigation

Tread the fine line between utility and humanity, whilst avoiding ageism. This is not a matter of 'investigate less' (or 'investigate more', although given the difficulty with diagnosis older people could be argued to need more access to high-tech investigation than younger people).

It is about weighing:
• Benefits (what you expect to get out of the test—information, potential treatment plans, both indicating and contra-indicating interventions).
• Burdens (the practicalities or unpleasantness of the test, possible complications or side effects).
• Autonomy or best interests (what the person wants, or would have wanted).

Blood tests 'come cheap'—make sure patients have an up-to-date full blood count, ESR, renal function and electrolytes, calcium, vitamin B12 and folate, and thyroid function. Use other tests to answer specific questions. Some still routinely test for syphilis serology in cognitive impairment, although tertiary syphilis is now vanishingly rare. Don't repeat tests done recently (B12 and thyroid function are not going to change over 6 months at least).

Beware tests that perform poorly as screening tests (i.e. in the absence of suggestive symptoms), such as prostate specific antigen (PSA) or carcino-embryonic antigen (CEA).

Other tests need more justification. In the absence of specific symptoms, we doubt the value of routine chest X-ray, but have a low threshold for requesting one (breathlessness, haemoptysis, chest pain, weight loss, finger clubbing).

CT head scanning for cognitive impairment is contentious (📖 Chapter 2, p. 38):
• Firstly, ensure that the test is achievable. An agitated or unco-operative patient is unlikely to yield a technically adequate scan. Sedation or anaesthesia is only justified if you have a specific question to answer. However, a modern CT scanner only takes a few minutes to acquire the images.
• The diagnostic yield is low (perhaps 1%) in delirium and dementia without focal neurological signs or other features like sustained drowsiness, headache, or seizures. However, the tragedy of missing a treatable pathology (subdural haematoma, tumour, hydrocephalus) might still be adequate justification.
• Scans are welcome (by carers and doctors) for the information they provide. The reassurance may be 'false' in the sense that treatable pathologies or tumours are rare, or usually cause other features that would prompt scanning.
• Evidence of large-vessel cerebrovascular disease may point towards a diagnosis of vascular dementia. However, you can neither diagnose dementia, nor its subtype, from a scan. Precise diagnosis is impossible ante-mortem. Cholinesterase inhibitor drugs are generally ineffective in vascular dementia. However, many reports of scans on older people describe 'chronic sub-cortical ischaemic change' (leukoariosis) which has an uncertain relationship to vascular dementia.

- Scanning is cheap—a fraction of the cost of a single day in hospital.
- In the UK, NICE recommends some form of imaging—CT is the easiest to achieve.

Some tests, such as barium enemas, are unpleasant, and you must be very sure that they are necessary and that alternatives are not possible. Get a specialty opinion or discuss with a radiologist.

Treatment

The best model for thinking about the range and type of intervention is the diagrammatic representation of the *WHO International Classification of Functioning, Disability and Health*, devised by Tormod Jaksholt (⊟ Figure 8.1).

Intervention should aim to:
• Prevent the preventable (including complications).
• Cure treatable pathologies.
• Palliate unpleasant symptoms.
• Remediate disabilities.
• Promote participation and reintegration.
• Be realistic and achievable.

A close specification of goals is vital. Much management in advanced dementia is 'primarily palliative'—more concerned with symptom control and maintenance of dignity and function than, for example, prevention.

Rehabilitation

The *Concise Oxford Dictionary* defines rehabilitation as 'A restoration to rights or former abilities.'

There are three elements:
• Re-ablement—restoration of function, reacquiring strength, stamina, dexterity, and cardio-respiratory fitness, taking advantage of sponta- neous recovery after acute illness, avoiding complications, learning new skills, and making use of aids and appliances.
• Resettlement—the adaptation of the environment to suit the abili- ties of the person concerned and maximize their participation. This includes family and other carer considerations, and their approach to ongoing support.
• Re-adjustment—psychological adaptation, changes in goals and ambi- tions, re-establishing esteem and fulfilment.

And two broad aims:
• To maximize functional ability.
• To increase the number of options that patients and their families have over eventual discharge—which often means making possible a home discharge where the alternative would have been institutional care.

However, in progressive diseases, and in dementia in particular, a further distinction is required, between 'restorative' and 'adaptive' rehabilitation.
• Restorative rehabilitation is centred on reacquiring lost functions (for example walking or regaining continence after a hip fracture or debili- tating acute illness). This may or may not be possible in people with dementia.
• Adaptive rehabilitation recognizes that independent performance of some functions will never be achieved, whereas supported perform- ance may be possible, for example in shopping or meal preparation.

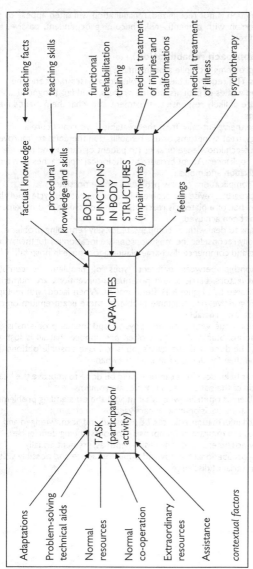

Fig. 8.1 Schematic representation of the WHO's framework for rehabilitation—the *International Classification of Functioning, Disability and Health* (ICF). The aim is to maximize activity and participation. Arrows represent necessary conditions. Devised by Dr Tormod Jaksholt.

If this distinction is not recognized, rehabilitation will often appear to fail, and the person with dementia risks becoming dependent, passive, and depersonalized.

How to approach rehabilitation

- Identify problems (compile a 'problem list').
- Set goals. This requires a blend of professional assessment and the views and wishes of patients and their carers, including prognostication, knowledge of likely response to treatment, and what the patient values and wants.
- Intervene therapeutically. Treat the treatable. If you can't cure a pathology, treat symptoms, or use rehabilitation therapies to improve function, teach knowledge or skills (to patient or carer), and provide aids and appliances. Adopt broadly 'psychological' approaches to maintain motivation and mood.
- Prevent complications or new problems where possible.
- Review progress, revise the problem list, and repeat the cycle until all goals are met, or a plateau is reached, when we assume that maximum ability has been achieved.
- Make plans to deal with, or compensate for, any remaining problems.
- Continually reconsider the most appropriate location for further management, and commence discharge planning for those in hospital.

The relationship between different types of problems is complex. Contextual factors, barriers, and potential interventions are numerous and complicated (☐ Figure 8.1). Be thorough. When faced with multiple, chronic, progressive, or intractable problems, there is a premium on correcting what is correctable.

A common issue with combined physical and mental problems is one of expectations. Staff and relatives often presuppose that all is lost and nothing can be done. The specialist's job is to make possible options that patients and their families did not think they had.

When all has been done that can or should be done to improve the health and function of the patient, analyse residual problems:

- The problem is often knowing what (if any) the outstanding problems are, and having decision-making paralysed by uncertainty.
- With hard information, risks can be assessed and acknowledged and plans made to mitigate or compensate for outstanding deficiencies.
- This may not be easy and requires in-depth assessment, usually involving occupational therapy and other therapists, and possibly visits home or a trial of discharge.

Problem lists

The problem list is a key tool in managing complex older patients:

* Identify, break down, and understand problems. This requires a thorough review of the case notes, discussion with the patient and family, and proper medical assessment and investigation.
* Make sure all problems are explained in terms of a diagnosis. Problems will often comprise a mix of physical, mental, and social issues. The term 'formulation' captures this better than simple 'diagnosis'.
* Over time, review diagnoses to ensure they are correct (the initial working diagnosis will often have to be revised in the light of progress, test results, and response to treatment).

'Problems' can be:

* A risk factor or predisposition.
* A diagnosis or pathology.
* An abnormal test result.
* An abnormality of body structure or function (impairment—often symptoms or examination findings).
* An inability to perform tasks or activities ('disabilities'), including difficult behaviours.
* Restricted participation—problems at the level of the person in a physical and social environment.
* A social issue (e.g. health of a carer, housing, relationships).

Cognitive problems take their place amongst other physical/medical and social issues. The activity/disability manifestation of cognitive problems will be behaviours—broadly including difficult behaviours (e.g. wandering, shouting) but also apathy and withdrawal, and the exercise of judgement and safety awareness.

Goal setting

Goals can be 'high level' (where you eventually want to get, for example, discharge home) or 'intermediate' (things that need to be achieved on the way to the higher level goals, such as walking or self-management of medicines).

Convene an early meeting with family, including the patient if he or she is able. Discuss:
- What they have already been told, and what they already know.
- Previous abilities, problems, and support.
- The diagnosis and its effects, especially on current abilities.
- Their expectations.
- The likely prognosis.
- Future options:
  - Keep all options open for as long as possible. Don't make any assumptions (e.g. that discharge to a care home will be inevitable).
  - Cover the likely duration of recovery and rehabilitation.
  - Broach the possibility of institutional discharge if it looks likely. Suggest that family members visit a few care homes. The local telephone directory is a good place to start, but in Britain the Commission for Social Care and Inspection website (www.csci. org.uk) may be more helpful. This enables future discussions to be better informed, and starts the process of finding a suitable home.

If the patient was previously living in a care home, useful information about previous abilities and goals (e.g. what abilities are required to enable a return to the previous home) can be gained by telephoning the home.

Multidisciplinary working

A range of approaches, techniques, and expertise is required to maximize the abilities of a frail older person and arrange suitable long-term support (📖 Table 8.2).

Table 8.2 Who does what? Roles of different members of the team

Who?	What?
Nurses	Observation, hygiene, basic nutrition, pressure area care, medication supervision, continence management, behavioural management, primary information point for family, continuity, practice of ADL skills, 24 h approach, discharge planning.
Physiotherapists	Assessment and training of motor function, remediation of mobility disabilities (including trunk control, bed mobility, transfers, walking, and stairs). Other specialist functions may include advice on orthoses, clearing secretions from the lungs, and teaching pelvic floor exercises.
Occupational therapists	Assessment and training in personal and domestic ADLs, seating and wheelchair assessment, home assessment visits, advising on and provision of aids and adaptations.
Speech and language therapists	Assessment and treatment of receptive and expressive language function. Communication training. Provision of communication aids. Advising families and other staff on communication. Support for dysphasic patients and their families. Assessment and management of neurogenic dysphagia.
Doctors	Compiling comprehensive medical formulation—diagnosis, including comorbidity, risk factors, and complications. Medical therapy and necessary specialist referral. Depending on local arrangements, co-ordination and overview, communication with patients and families.
Dieticians	Assessment of nutritional needs and recommendations on specialist diets (including cholesterol and weight reduction). Planning of tube feeding regimens.
Clinical psychologists	Assessment of cognitive impairments, perceptual disorders, executive functions (planning, decision-making), mood disorders, anxiety, adjustment reactions, and emotionalism. Explanation to patients, carers, and clinical staff. Direct clinical interventions include cognitive retraining, group or individual psychotherapy, behaviour management, relaxation, and cognitive behavioural therapy. Supportive counselling and groups for carers.
Social workers	Mainly discharge planning: need for home care support services, meals at home, day centres, and institutional care, including respite care. Advice and assessment for financial benefits and institutional care funding. Also may help with suspected abuse, debt counselling, guardianship, and MHA orders.

Teamwork

- A team is a group of people working together with a common purpose.
- Teams achieve more than individuals working in isolation.
- Each team member should know what they bring to the team, their skills and limitations, and what they are responsible for. Doctors in particular should not forget that it is their job to get the medicine (and psychiatry) right (diagnosis, drug therapy, referral to other specialists).
- Team members should know what other members do. There will be some overlap, but unnecessary replication should be avoided.
- The team should follow the same approach and strategy 24 h a day, regardless of which discipline they are from.
- Communication is essential, usually via weekly team meetings, when patients are systematically reviewed for problems, abilities, progress towards goals, and when new goals are set and discharge planning undertaken.
- Each involved team member needs to contribute to meetings—and be helped to do so if reticent.
- An objective record of disabilities should be kept, by using standardized scales, or free text.
- Records should be shared or easily accessible to all team members.
- Leadership of health care teams tends to be quite informal—meetings need chairing or directing, but decisions are a matter of consensus, and delegation requires persuasion rather than giving orders (📖 Box 8.1).

Box 8.1 Leadership and teamwork

- Leaders:
  - Leaders do not just give orders, but enable people to do their jobs better.
  - Team members enable their leaders to lead, because it is in their interests, makes it easier for them to do their own jobs, and helps to achieve a worthwhile common goal.
- Leadership functions:
  - integrating information
  - maintaining momentum
  - helping set goals
  - making or confirming decisions
  - developing a vision, identifying new opportunities.
- Teamwork needs:
  - clear and agreed roles and duties
  - equal commitment
  - shared responsibility
  - identification and use of individuals' strengths
  - clear communication and sharing of information
  - honest, constructive feedback, including thanks and praise
  - mutual support (e.g. when things go wrong).

Rehabilitation nursing

There are two complimentary nursing roles, one or other of which may predominate but which often go together:
- Supportive, active, 'doing for' care, in severe acute illness (acute nursing).
- Encouraging, enabling, progressive withdrawal of support to promote independence (rehabilitation nursing).

Rehabilitation nursing may be the single most important element of a rehabilitation unit, requiring flexibility and fine judgement. It is often under-recognized, including by patients and relatives, who expect to be 'cared for'. It involves:
- Using opportunities during daily care to undertake functional activities (getting up, toileting, dressing, walking to the day room or to meals).
- The progressive withdrawal of support as independence and confidence are regained.

This is achieved through:
- Practise of skills or approaches learned with rehabilitation therapists, and avoidance of inappropriate activities.
- Building of stamina, fitness, and confidence through physical activity.
- Avoidance of complications (pressure sores, joint contractures, venous thrombosis, aspiration, falls).
- Implementing behaviour management plans consistently.
- Making specialist assessments and management plans for continence and wound care.
- Providing detailed feedback on day to day performance.
- Helping to formulate, and working towards, defined goals.
- Providing sufficient help to ensure 'personal maintenance' (hygiene, nutrition, freedom from falls and other dangers).
- Being aware of general health, and the ability to react appropriately in a medical crisis.
- Helping to promote psychological adjustment (listening, advising, promoting a positive outlook).
- Being aware of and managing patients' and relatives' expectations, in particular where this is manifest as dysfunctional illness behaviour (such as over-dependency or over-protectiveness), or over-optimistic goals.

Monitoring progress

Progress is best monitored by assessing disability (activity limitation). Three key dimensions are:

- Mobility—transfers, walking, stability and falls, getting to the toilet, stairs, wheelchair use. Include distance achieved and extent of help and aids required (e.g. walks 20 m with a wheeled Zimmer frame plus one person).
- Continence—and other practical elimination issues such as constipation, nocturia, and urinary urgency.
- Behaviour—usually in the context of dementia or a difficult pre-morbid personality trait, but also mood, motivation, engagement, and passivity.

Other aspects such as washing and dressing, kitchen skills, outdoor mobility, money management, and visiting a shop should be added at the appropriate stage of rehabilitation.

In hospital, a standardized activities of daily living scale (e.g. Bristol ADL scale/Barthel Index, 📖 Chapter 13) can be used. Ensure sufficient annotation to record the presumed mechanism of outstanding problems. Is the transfer difficulty due to cognition, weakness, pain, dizziness, or fear? This may prompt a medical review.

Once home, a wider range of activities should be considered.

Preventing delirium

Delirium is not always avoidable, but some evidence demonstrates that its new onset in hospital is not immutable.

A large American randomized trial found that a structured, if labour-intensive, daily programme addressing orientation, sleep, vision, hearing, mobility, and hydration reduced the incidence of delirium by a third amongst at-risk individuals.

In some cases the onset of delirium reflects bad medical and nursing practice. Doing simple things thoroughly and correctly minimizes risk. In particular, attention to drug prescribing, avoiding polypharmacy and especially common culprit drugs (antimuscarinic, opiates), avoidance of infection risks (urinary catheters, aspiration), venous thromboembolism, and hypoxia. Equally important is the prompt detection and diagnosis of medical problems (infections, metabolic disturbance, heart failure) as early treatment will minimize delirium risk and time spent in delirium (□ Box 3.3 p. 71).

Models of liaison psychiatry

Shared care ward

There are only a few of these, in the UK at least. They are staffed with both physical and mental health medical, nursing, and therapy staff. They aim to improve process and outcome of care by:

- Early accurate diagnosis.
- Optimal medical and psychiatric management, avoiding neuroleptic medication if possible, and making the most appropriate choices of drugs if not.
- Early meetings with families and carers, defining expectations, giving explanation, and goal setting.
- Close links with community mental health teams, intermediate care, specialist intensive dementia home support, and care homes.
- Improved risk management (more willingness to take risks on home discharges).

Time can be saved if accurate assessment is completed early, and early engagement made with families and carers on expectation and goals. For example if there is no will to return home, planning for care home placement can begin without delay. On the other hand, even if ambitious goals for home discharge are identified early, early links can be made with community services, possibly avoiding a lengthy wait for a care home placement. The idea is to have systems in place that optimize care and avoid delays.

Peripatetic liaison service

For working age adults and children, there are well-established liaison services. They adopt a peripatetic consultation model, with consultant or trainee psychiatrists or liaison nurses making assessments, giving advice (usually on drug treatment), and offering some outpatient assessment or follow-up.

Similar services for older people are rare. This is partly because many medical geriatricians have some expertise in managing mental health problems in older people and will necessarily have close working relationships with old-age psychiatrists. However, links with these services and community mental health teams can be patchy, and patients on general medical or surgical wards can miss out.

An alternative working model is for assessments to be made by a liaison mental health nurse. They need support from a consultant psychiatrist (or interested physician).

In general, the evidence supporting peripatetic services is not good, but mostly comes from other disciplines (stroke, general geriatric medicine). There is some evidence that peripatetic delirium consultation can reduce length of stay and improve outcomes, and that liaison nurses can improve the process of care, if not the outcome.

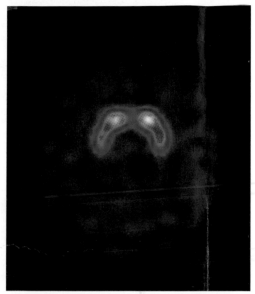

Plate 1 Normal appearance of DaTSCAN®.

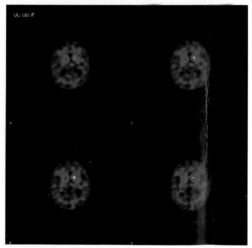

Plate 2 DaTSCAN® in a case of dementia with Lewy bodies, showing reduced uptake of isotope into the caudate nuclei. (Courtesy of GE Healthcare).

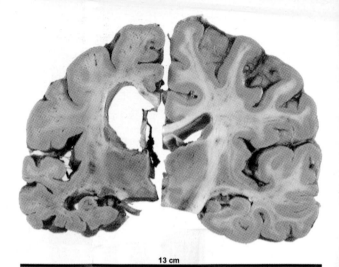

Plate 3 Composite plate showing section through brain of a case of severe Alzheimer's Disease (left) and normal control (right).

13 cm

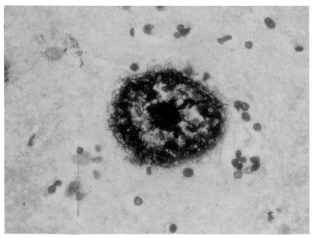

Plate 4 Neuritic plaque.

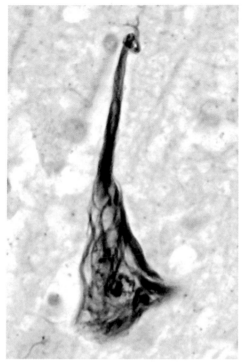

Plate 5 Neurofibrillary Tangle.

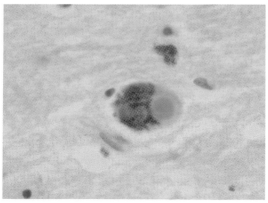

Plate 6 Cortical Lewy body.

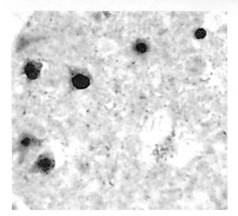

Plate 7 Pick bodies stained to demonstrate τ protein.

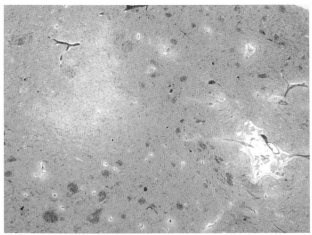

Plate 8 Vascular dementia showing lacunar infarct (left) and arteriosclerosis (right).

Elective admission of people with dementia

The risks are:
- Failure to identify the comorbidity.
- Inability to gain consent for interventions and operations.
- Assumptions about understanding, abilities, and coping resources at home.
- Development of delirium as a complication to the interventions, as a result of anaesthetic, opiate analgesics (codeine and dihydrocodeine are notorious culprits), night sedatives, complicating infection, heart attack, stroke, or venous thromboembolism.
- Behavioural decompensation (unfamiliar environment and routine).

Surgeons, anaesthetists, and nursing and therapy staff must be aware of the possibility of dementia as a comorbidity, and delirium as a possible complication.

The key is close communication and careful planning with family and carers, close observation to spot potential problems, and requesting appropriate and responsive medical, geriatric, or psychiatric advice when there are problems.

People with dementia and delirium are likely to take longer to recover than the cognitively intact. At the same time they stand to lose most by unnecessarily prolonged hospital stays. Each hospital requires a system for identifying these problems and asking for appropriate help quickly (liaison psychiatry, old-age psychiatry or mental health nursing, geriatricians, or other discharge facilitation schemes).

Issues of decision-making, consent, and assessment of best interests are covered elsewhere (📖 Chapters 11 and 12).

Confusion in the A&E department

There are three main scenarios, and each needs proper identification, assessment, understanding, and planning:

- Medical emergency, accident, or injury.
- Behavioural emergency.
- Social emergency.

It will never be easy to undertake this in an emergency department; sometimes it will be impossible.

Issues include:

- This represents a high risk situation—assessment of severity of acute and chronic illness, usual and current functional abilities, and support resources is difficult, especially given time pressure, skill set, and physical environment of an emergency department.
- Disturbed behaviour may need pharmacological control to allow any sort of medical assessment (but this may itself make subsequent assessment difficult).
- Accessing alternative services for assessment and help is difficult at short notice—e.g. secondary care psychiatry, community mental health, intermediate care, or social services home care.
- You can help follow-on services by taking as much of a history, especially third party history, as possible. More importantly, make sure that contact details for relatives or carers are clearly recorded so that later contact can be made.
- Commonly, and quite correctly, these situations will lead to emergency medical admission, if only to provide a place of safety in a crisis, observation, and medical and mental health assessment. Such admissions may be resented by medical teams with little expertise and sympathy for the problems, and the feeling that they are not their responsibility.
- Beware things that can make matters worse:
  - over-sedation (especially in delirium or dementia with Lewy bodies)
  - confrontation
  - opiate analgesia
  - falling off trolleys, fractures
  - careless comments about the inappropriateness of the admission (hardly the fault of the patient or worried family), the actions of other professionals (such as GPs), and the need for care home placement (you cannot decide this until a full assessment has been made)
  - dehydration, starvation, or pressure sores
  - urinary catheterization
  - omission of regular drugs.

Discharge

Discharge

The time for hospital discharge is when what is needed can be provided elsewhere. Much nursing and rehabilitation can be delivered at home. Increasingly, community services are available that can do this. However, discharging someone with moderate or severe dementia who lives alone remains a major challenge.

Is discharge safe?

Consider fitness for discharge at the levels of:
- The person.
- Their abilities.
- The environment.

At the person level, this will mean being 'medically stable':
- In a stable cardiac rhythm, with adequate blood pressure, free from severe heart failure or any life-threatening cardiovascular problems (acute coronary syndrome, tamponade).
- Adequate, and stable, respiratory function.
- Free from acute renal failure or other severe metabolic derangement such as severe dehydration or electrolyte or glucose disturbance.
- Free from severe infection.
- Able to swallow safely, or having a means of non-oral feeding (i.e. a PEG tube).
- Free from severe debilitating symptoms such as frequent fits, pain, nausea, or breathlessness.

At the level of activities, at a minimum, it will require:
- Ability to transfer from bed to chair, wheelchair, or commode, alone or with a willing and able carer (with a hoist if necessary).
- Continence or adequate containment.
- Measures to relieve skin pressure.
- Ability, judgement, and insight to avoid falls, injury, or other safety problems (or appropriate supervision).
- Ability to take prescribed drugs, or someone to supervise them.

The environment divides into the physical and social environment:
- Sufficient human help—full-time, if help may be required urgently or unpredictably; otherwise sufficient to ensure:
  - toileting
  - pressure area care
  - feeding and hygiene
  - occupation
  - safety from falls or other injury
  - social and emotional contact.
- Adequate equipment, including:
  - suitable bed and chair
  - pressure relieving mattresses and cushions
  - commode, urinals, or bedpan
  - feeding equipment (e.g. feeding pumps for PEG feeds)
  - pendant alarm or mobile phone if left alone for periods of time
  - means of entry for care staff if living alone (key safe or door entry system)

- mobility aids (wheelchair, sticks, or frame; rotunda, sliding board, or hoist for transfers)
- rails to facilitate bed and toilet transfers.

Exceptions:
- In some cases, such as discharge for home terminal care, safety (in terms of protecting life) is not a prime concern. But many of the same considerations are needed to make the discharge practical and humane.
- Hospital is not a prison. Patients cannot be detained unless they consent, or have been shown to lack capacity and remaining in hospital is in their best interests (☐ Chapter 11). Remember that capacity must be assumed unless it can be demonstrated otherwise.
- Health and safety legislation applies to care staff. They cannot therefore undertake tasks carrying undue risk—for example manual transfers represent a risk of back injury and a hoist may be required. If the patient refuses a hoist or there is no room in a cramped bedroom, and alternative arrangements cannot be made, staff cannot be expected to undertake transfers. Other sources of risk include aggressive or disinhibited patients with cognitive impairment.

Is appropriate community support and follow-up available?

Community support divides into restorative services (trying to improve function) and prosthetic or adaptive services (making up for things the person cannot do themselves).

Restorative services include:
- Community mental health teams.
- Early discharge support and rehabilitation teams.
- Day hospitals.
- Generic community services such as family doctors, district nursing, community physiotherapy, Social Services occupational therapy (who are responsible for providing many aids and home adaptations), and speech and language therapy.
- Models of 'intermediate care' based in residential or nursing homes, possibly with access to frequent in-the-home rehabilitation whilst still providing 24 h (especially overnight) supervision.

Prosthetic services include:
- Social Services home care, including help to get up and go to bed, with washing and dressing, getting meals, emptying catheter bags or commodes, supervising medication, housework, and shopping.
- Meals at home service (from Social Services or private equivalents, or someone to buy 'ready meals' at the supermarket and a microwave to heat them in).
- Day centres.
- Visitor and advocate schemes.
- Sitting services for carers.
- Respite care in residential or nursing homes.
- Permanent placement in a residential or nursing home.

Both types of service must be aware of the need for 'adaptive rehabilitation' providing supported performance where full independence cannot be regained.

Are the carers prepared?

The presence of a willing carer can enable a discharge that would otherwise be impossible.

Such carers:
- Provide hands-on care, in much the same way as Social Services home care—transferring, toileting, catheter care and changing pads, getting meals, other domestic tasks, operating feeding pumps for PEG tubes, giving medication.
- Provide supervision and surveillance (looking out for problems).
- Provide company, occupation, and emotional support.

The commitment of some carers, and the range of tasks they will take on, can be staggering. Many of these are tasks that previous everyday life has not prepared them for, such as:
- Changing wet or soiled incontinence pads.
- Safe transfers (safe for both patient and carer), or operating a hoist.
- Supervised walking.
- Dressing.
- Feeding, sometimes for people with precarious swallowing, who need advice on positioning, consistencies, and pacing of feeds.
- Pressure area care, including turning, and operating pressure relieving mattresses.
- Administration of medicines, including insulin.
- Catheter care.
- Intermittent urinary catheterization.

These needs should be anticipated during rehabilitation and carers should be given appropriate training by OT, physiotherapy, and nursing staff.

Elderly partners are often frail themselves. Statutory services may be required to support an 'informal' carer:
- In the UK they have a statutory right to have their own needs assessed by Social Services departments.
- Respite care (a period in a residential or nursing home, or sometimes a hospital, to give carers a holiday or break) may need to be anticipated and arranged. However, moving someone with cognitive impairment from one location to another can be unsettling for patients and upsetting for carers, who may consider such 'respite' more trouble than it is worth.
- Sitting services can allow a carer a few hours to go shopping or to pursue social or leisure activities of their own. Opportunities for these can become very limited when caring for a very dependent person.
- Night sitting services can be valuable to help someone manage when nights are disturbed. But access is limited from statutory services and cost is high if arranged privately.

Is the environment optimized?

Environments can facilitate activity and participation, or provide a barrier to it. Examples include access ramps, stair rails or stair lifts, grab rails around toilets and baths, bathing equipment such as bath boards, 'glide about' chairs (with wheels on) for use in a shower, or 'bed leavers' (a rail by the bed supported under the mattress).

Wheelchair users will need sufficient space to manoeuvre, doors that are wide enough to get through, and toilets with enough space to allow safe transfers. Kitchen work surfaces may need to be lower to allow use.

Home visits by occupational therapists, with or without the patient, a physiotherapist, members of the patient's family, and representatives of Social Services, are immensely useful. They serve several purposes:

- An assessment of the physical environment, to look for hazards and other barriers.
- To plan therapeutic changes to the environment (ramps and rails, replacing or altering beds and chairs, recommending improved lighting, removal of clutter, loose wires, and rugs, acquiring kitchen aids).
- Assessing the patient's performance of tasks in the home environment.
- Assessing the viability of community rehabilitation.
- To motivate and encourage the patient, as a clear indication that progress is being made and discharge planning is taking place.
- To boost the confidence of patient and family or other carers, not least by showing that proper planning is taking place.
- To demonstrate that someone will not manage at home, especially if there is dispute about this (whilst realizing safety is a relative and graded phenomenon, not absolute, and that a single home visit will never give a definitive assessment).

Alternative assessment opportunities include:

- Trial periods in a 'rehabilitation flat' attached to a rehabilitation unit. This can be alone or with a carer such as a spouse. Routine professional input is limited to what a home-care package might provide.
- Overnight stay at home.
- 'Weekend leave' (i.e. several nights).

Summary

1. For various (mostly legitimate) reasons, confused people form a large part of the workload of general hospitals. Hospitals can provide a valuable and productive role in addressing the problems presented, although there are many challenges.

2. Assessment must be thorough, usually multidisciplinary, and take account of function and social issues as well as diagnosis. However, do not forget the crucial role of diagnosis in defining the contribution of medicine to problems presented by older people. Multiple pathology and non-specific presentations are to be expected.

3. The management approach is broadly rehabilitative, by which we mean restoring function, optimizing the environment, and resetting expectations. In dementia, adaptation or support to maintain roles and abilities is also important.

4. Ideally, dedicated services should be commissioned for older people with combined medical and mental health problems. Other models of peripatetic liaison can also be useful.

5. Elective admissions and A&E attendances are occasions of special risk and concern.

6. Careful discharge planning is required, but keep all options (including that of returning home) open for as long as possible.

Chapter 9

217

'Physical' problems in dementia

What is the issue?

Why treat people with dementia differently? In many respects you can manage physical problems in someone who happens to have dementia exactly as you would in anyone else.

However:
- People with dementia often have comorbid physical problems.
- Sometimes it is the 'physical' disorder that causes most problems (incontinence, falls).
- Dementia is a risk factor for some of these problems (incontinence, immobility, falls).
- Behaviour problems and a lack of insight and judgement can contribute to the 'physical' problems.
- Reliable and safe taking of medication is uncertain.
- Assessment can be complicated by the presence of dementia:
  - reporting of symptoms is more unreliable
  - tests may not be understood or tolerated as well, or may be deemed unduly burdensome.
- Therapies that require new learning may not be as effective, and a different approach may be required.

Problems with medication

Clinical therapeutics

It is not uncommon to see patients admitted to hospital taking 10 or 15 different drugs. Evidence suggests that compliance on the fourth drug is 50% (amongst the cognitively intact). But you never know which the fourth drug is.

Starting and stopping drugs is one of the easiest things doctors do, but is not necessarily done well. As a general rule, check:

- Indication: make sure each drug has a good indication. Approach this critically—review case notes, phone the GP. Ask:
  - Who made the diagnosis?
  - On what evidence? Diuretics, statins, antiparkinsonian drugs, and antidepressants often lack a clear indication, and a 'stopping trial' may be required (stop it and see if the problem re-emerges). But don't be cavalier. If a neurologist diagnosed Parkinson's disease, or a cardiologist heart failure, then most likely they are right.
  - Is there evidence that a therapeutic (as opposed to preventative) drug has been reviewed for effect?
- Drug choice: make sure the most suitable drug is being used. Consider:
  - efficacy (however, comparative efficacy studies are often not available)
  - potential side effects
  - duration of action (once a day is convenient, but accumulation may be a problem e.g. glibenclamide, benzodiazepines)
  - generics are usually cheaper, and the advantages of newer over older drugs are sometimes overstated.
- Concordance: make sure there is a reasonable chance that prescribed drugs are actually taken, and taken correctly.
- Review for problems and efficacy. This can be difficult (it is essentially an uncontrolled observation, both for effects and side effects). Make sure the drug has been titrated up to the optimal dose. You may need to stop and restart if unsure whether a particular symptom is a drug side effect.
  - Beware of using one drug to counter the side effects of another (although there are exceptions, for example co-prescribing proton pump inhibitors and non-steroidal anti-inflammatory drugs).
  - Side effects caused by preventative drugs are rarely justified (antihypertensives, anti-thrombotics, anticoagulants, cholesterol lowering drugs, osteoporosis drugs). You cause a problem now to prevent something that may never happen—and the odds are usually that it will never happen.
- Balance likely benefits with risks and burdens. Use the decision-making framework (📖 Chapter 12). Negotiate with the patient and carers. For example warfarin is a dangerous drug but potent at preventing embolic complications of atrial fibrillation, mitral stenosis, and left ventricular dysfunction. Decisions on its use must be made case-by-case, without overemphasizing benefits or underemphasizing risks. But don't make presumptions, for example on how an individual balances these, or on compliance if this is going to be closely supervised.

- The concept of a periodic medication review is important, perhaps every 6 months as a minimum, and usually undertaken in primary care (who have responsibility for long-term prescribing in the UK).
- Beware of stopping drugs suddenly—sometimes there will be withdrawal effects (opiates, benzodiazepines, SSRIs).
- If drugs are unlikely to be taken reliably:
  - care professionals should know
  - deliberately choose which drugs (usually no more than one or two) are most important and abandon the rest.
- If you stop or start drugs during a hospital admission, especially an unusual drug or one used for an unusual indication, explicitly tell the GP in the discharge summary or clinic letter so that stopped drugs are not inadvertently restarted, or useful drugs stopped during a routine drug review.
- Know if a particular drug is prone to side effects and find out if those effects are occurring (🔲 Box 9.1).
- Develop a relatively restricted personal formulary of drugs you know very well. This will often be guided by hospital or other policies (for example local formularies or preferred prescribing lists). You may have to look outside this list when particular problems or other circumstances arise.

Concordance/compliance

Help improve compliance if you can:
- Simplify the drug regimen as far as possible:
  - be sure that each drug is necessary
  - use once-a-day drugs or formulations whenever possible
  - If a non-resident carer is needed to supervise medication this will usually have to be a morning dose (or ask when is most convenient)
  - use fixed-dose combinations if these are available and suitable.
- Make remembering what tablets to take and when as easy as possible:
  - Enlist support from relatives to supervise tablet taking. Negotiations on supervision of medication may have to be opened early.
  - If possible encourage patients to understand their drugs, know what they are for, and when to take them. Nurses and pharmacists can help here. If a relative is going to supervise, advise them similarly.
  - Explain drug changes as you make them. Some patients are bemused and upset by apparently random stopping and starting of drugs on ward rounds.
  - Self-administration of drugs whilst in hospital helps with familiarity, gives practice, and can alert staff to patients who cannot take drugs reliably.
  - On discharge, write down what to take when.
  - Use 'dosette' boxes or commercial blister pack services (from retail pharmacists—at a cost) if necessary.
  - Social Services home care will often prompt to take tablets, but will not usually administer them.
  - You can assume that people in residential or nursing homes will have medication administered reliably.
- Patients may not be able to open child-resistant containers. Check, and provide alternatives if necessary.

Adverse effects

Adverse effects of drugs:

- Increase with age due to age- or disease-related changes in drug metabolism and pharmacokinetics, co-morbidities, drug interactions, and compliance.
- Some are obvious (e.g. dry mouth with antimuscarinic medication), and are common enough to spot at the individual patient level.
- Others are more subtle—if you give a drug to very large numbers of people, a small increase in risk can increase incidence of a disease at a population level, although each individual's chances of being affected are very small. NSAIDs (peptic ulceration), antipsychotics (stroke or arrhythmia), antipsychotics and antidepressants (falls) are examples. By the same measure, many preventative drugs reduce incidence at the population level but are unlikely to benefit the individual. Aspirin in vascular disease prevents one event per 78 person-years of taking, so most people who take aspirin do not benefit from it. Yet at the population level this will prevent 1000 strokes a year.
- Know the common ones (📖 Box 9.1).

Box 9.1 Common adverse effects of drugs

By drug
- Antipsychotics—drowsiness, extrapyramidal effects (even atypicals), falls, impotence, galactorrhoea.
- Benzodiazepines—drowsiness, falls, cognitive slowing or impairment, withdrawal effects.
- Antimuscarinic—delirium, dry mouth, urinary retention, blurred vision, dyspepsia, constipation.
- Tricyclic antidepressants—antimuscarinic, drowsiness, falls.
- Diuretics—lower urinary tract symptoms, dehydration, hyponatraemia, hypokalaemia, hyperglycaemia, gout.
- Antihypertensives, antianginals, anti-arrhythmics—hypotension (especially postural), heart failure.
- Antiparkinsonian—delirium, hypotension, dyskinesia, nausea.
- Lithium—polyuria, tremor.
- Antiepileptic drugs—drowsiness, cognitive slowing or impairment, ataxia.

By adverse effect
- Delirium—antimuscarinic (including tricyclic antidepressant, antiparkinsonian, surgical premedication, bladder instability drugs, disopyramide), opiates.
- Diarrhoea—laxatives, antibiotics, metformin, proton pump inhibitors, NSAIDs.
- Hypotension—diuretics, all other cardiovascular drugs except digoxin, levodopa, antipsychotics.
- Falls—sedative and antidepressant drugs (TCA and SSRI), hypnotics, drugs causing hypotension.
- Rash, pruritus—any.

Dizzy spells and falls

Falls, and fear of falling, are common and limiting. Half or more of people with dementia fall each year. Remember that falls are inevitable if mobility is encouraged—a complete absence of falls suggests an undue restriction on mobility.

Consequences

- 10–20% of falls result in injuries.
- 5% result in fractures.
- 1% result in hip fractures, the most feared consequence.
- Loss of confidence.
- Restricted activities.
- Unwillingness to walk outside or on stairs.
- Need for additional human help or supervision.
- Institutionalization.

Understand the balance system

Four mechanisms detect sway or postural instability:
- Vision.
- The vestibular system.
- Proprioception in the neck and legs.
- Tactile sensation in the feet.

The motor (pyramidal, extrapyramidal, and cerebellar) and musculo-skeletal systems provide the mechanism for adjusting to perturbations. Central processing, in particular reaction time, connects the two. But balance is not just static (e.g. standing still). Posture has to be maintained during walking, climbing stairs, and other activities. Hence anticipation, sequencing, planning, and judgement are also required. Any (or several) of these may be abnormal due to dementia, comorbidity, or deconditioning.

Causes of falls

Falls can be classified in several different ways:
- By main cause (about a third each):
  - 'acute' illness (pneumonia, arrhythmia, stroke, gastro-intestinal bleed, metabolic or electrolyte disturbance). Falling is one of the 'geriatric giants'—the non-specific presentations of any illness in an older person.
  - 'chronic' illness (in particular chronic neurological disease, including dementia; arthritis; visual problems)
  - environmental (accidents, tripping, lighting).
- Predisposition and precipitation:
  - Anyone can fall. What varies is the chance that any given activity, pathophysiological or environmental insult will result in failure to maintain balance, and the likelihood of a resulting injury.
  - A long list of risk factors has been described, some of which are modifiable (📖 Table 9.1). The more risk factors there are, the greater the chance of falling—so interventions tend to be multifac-torial, to remove or reduce as many risk factors as possible.

- The precipitant may or may not be obvious. A single adequate explanation (syncope, acute stroke, heart attack, pulmonary embolus, trauma, tripping, misjudgement) should be sought, but will often be uncertain.
- Syncopal or non-syncopal, presence or absence of dizziness (📖 Table 9.2):
  - syncope (loss of consciousness) has particular diagnostic implications that must be recognized (head trauma, cardiovascular, epileptic, hypoglycaemic)
  - unfortunately, syncope is often associated with amnesia for the event (in 30% of cases in the otherwise cognitively intact).
- Injurious/non-injurious—may give clues to mechanism and be helpful in risk assessment:
  - loss of consciousness
  - presence of protective reactions.
- Dizziness may give diagnostic clues—there are three main types:
  - Presyncope—'light headedness, as if about to faint', blurred or darkened vision, possibly bilateral tinnitus. Commonly experienced standing up from a hot bath. Generally implies cardiovascular causes (📖 Table 9.2).
  - Vertigo—spinning or hallucination of other relative movement between the person and the environment. Implies vestibular or brainstem dysfunction.
  - Dysequilibrium—the perception of unsteadiness, more non-specific, but may be neurological or musculo-skeletal in origin. A brief (few seconds) dysequilibrium ensues when the (arthritic) neck is extended during standing.

Table 9.1 Main risk factors for falls (predisposition)

Factor	Approximate relative risk
Age	1.5 per 10 years
Previous falls (any in previous year)	2.5
Acute illness	5
Dementia	2.5
Depression	1.5
Parkinson's disease	5
Stroke	4
Lower limb arthritis	2
Proximal muscle weakness	2–3
Abnormal gait	2.5
Housebound	2.5
History of heart disease	1.5
Postural hypotension	2
Taking 4 or more prescription drugs	2
Sedative, neuroleptic, or antidepressant medication	3
Hypotensive medication (antihypertensives, diuretics, antianginals, anti-arrhythmics)	1.5
Poor vision	2
Foot problems	1.5

Table 9.2 Causes of syncope and presyncope

Factor	Comment	Intervention
Head trauma	Usually obvious, look for lacerations, beware cervical spine injury	Supportive. CT if suspected intra-cranial bleeding (drowsy, features of raised intra-cranial pressure, focal neurology).
Epilepsy	Generalized seizures. Get a description from a witness. Ask about ictal and post-ictal features.	Investigate cause. Antiepileptic drugs, start with sodium valproate.
Intra-cranial bleeding	Intracerebral or subarachnoid haemorrhage. Highly unlikely to be transient unless it precipitates a seizure.	CT. Supportive acute management, rehabilitation, or terminal care.
Hypoglycaemia	Loss of consciousness only if severe, unless it precipitates a seizure	Intravenous 50 ml 20% glucose; intramuscular glucagon
Vasovagal syncope	3Ps—provocation, posture, prodrome	Reassurance, advice
Postural hypotension	Usually due to drugs, also autonomic neuropathy, or age-related autonomic dysfunction	Minimize culprit drugs; compression hosiery; fludrocortisone, midodrine
Carotid sinus hypersensitivity	Cardio-inhibitory and vasodepressor types; diagnosed on tilt testing	Pacemaker, advice, drug trial
Other provoked syncopes	Micturition, defaecation, cough	Advice
Brady-arrhythmias	Heart block, Stokes-Adams attacks, sick sinus syndrome	Pacemaker
Tachy-arrhythmias	Sustained or paroxysmal AF, SVT, VT	Anti-arrhythmic drugs
Tight aortic stenosis	Typically exertional syncope (but uncommon)	Surgery if otherwise fit
Acute myocardial infarction	Temporary or permanent myocardial damage and pump failure; provoked transient arrhythmia; vasovagal secondary to pain	Supportive in the first instance

Falls assessment

Most helpful is the predisposition and precipitant model:
- First explain the fall (unexplained falls may be due to syncope with amnesia).
- Then identify what risk factors make this individual more or less prone to fall.

To explain the fall, ask 'What happened?' 'How did you come to fall?' The question 'Do you remember hitting the floor?' may help exclude syncope, but it is not very reliable and will be even more compromised with chronic memory impairment.

You always need a history from a witness if there is syncope or an unexplained fall, and almost always if there is memory impairment and no syncope:
- What were the circumstances of the fall? What was the patient doing? Sitting, standing, lying? Was there a clear and sufficient cause (tripping, being pushed, falling out of bed, standing without habitually-required supervision)?
- Was there any warning? Did the patient complain of feeling dizzy? Was there time to sit down? Or did the patient fall to the ground? Distinguish between presyncope (light headedness as if about to faint); vertigo (spinning); dysequilibrium (unsteadiness because you are unsteady, as if drunk).
- What did they look like? Cardiovascular causes often cause a 'deathly pallor'—a compensatory surge of adrenaline and sympathetic activity shuts down the skin blood vessels. Generalized epilepsy causes transient respiratory arrest, and the patient may go blue. Convulsions, tongue biting, or incontinence may be evident.
- Were there associated symptoms such as chest pain or breathlessness? Or ear symptoms such as (new) deafness, pain, tinnitus, or discharge?
- Did anyone take the pulse?
- Has this happened before? If so, how often? Are there dizzy spells that do not lead to syncope? Are there obvious precipitants?
- Take a drug history. Is there anything recently started? Is acute or chronic alcohol excess involved?
- Assess general function, including transfers, walking, stairs, outdoor mobility, dressing, and bladder function (hurrying to the toilet can lead to lapses of judgement; nocturia is another occasion of risk).

Examination during a syncopal episode is invaluable, especially pulse, blood pressure (ECG rhythm strip if available), respiratory rate, or neurological signs (tone, plantar responses).

Between attacks a thorough cardiovascular, neurological, musculo-skeletal, and ear examination is required:
- Pulse rate, rhythm, and character. Check blood pressure after 5 minutes lying down, then after 30 seconds, 1 minute, and 3 minutes standing (preferably using an automated machine—remembering that these can take a good 20 seconds to make a recording). Pulse character is prolonged and volume is low in tight aortic stenosis, but this is difficult for inexperienced practitioners to assess reliably.

- Examine for heart murmurs, suggesting aortic stenosis or other structural abnormalities such as hypertrophic cardiomyopathy. Get an echocardiogram if suspicious.
- Test visual acuity (separately in each eye) and examine for cataracts. Are the spectacles up to date? Make a pin hole (14G needle through an X-ray request card). Re-examine the acuity looking through the pin hole. If it is better, the spectacle prescription needs reviewing.
- Test visual fields, and for visual inattention. Examine for Parkinsonism (cogwheel rigidity, best felt at the wrist), bradykinesia (touch the thumb on each finger in turn), and tremor. Examine for pyramidal (upper motor neurone) lesions—weakness, increased tone and reflexes, upgoing plantar responses. Pronator drift (hold the hands outstretched for 20 seconds, fingers facing up, fingers spread, eyes shut) is a sensitive test for subtle weakness. Also test proximal muscle power (shoulder abduction, hip flexion) and for lower limb sensation loss (pin prick, vibration, proprioception). Test for tactile inattention (touch left then right then both sides together. Perception of touch on the abnormal side is suppressed when there is a competing stimulus on the other side). You can also use Albert's test (line cancellation) or clock drawing (□ Chapter 13) to assess hemispatial neglect. Test cerebellar function (finger-nose ataxia, dysdiadochokinesia—clumsiness on rapid repeated movements).
- Examine the neck—cervical spondylosis is associated with a short-lived (few seconds) dizziness, especially on standing up or looking up (when the neck extends). This is due to malfunctioning proprioception (the old story about vertebrobasilar ischaemia is false). Hip and knee arthritis can cause unsteadiness either due to mechanical instability or nociceptive inhibition (painful joints inhibit the muscles supporting them, giving sudden loss of supporting tone around an acutely painful joint). Examine the feet for overgrown toenails (onychogryphosis), corns and calluses, ulcers, and other deformities.
- Check hearing, examine the tympanic membranes, and do Romberg's test (stand unsupported, feet shoulder-width apart, eyes shut, maintain for 20 seconds; if the patient takes a step to maintain balance the test is positive). If vertigo is described lying down, the diagnosis is likely to be benign paroxysmal positional vertigo. The Dix-Hallpike test may help (lie the patient from sitting with the head slightly extended over the end of an examination couch. Passively rotate the neck to one side, and in a separate test, the other). Keep eyes open. Symptoms may be reproduced. Nystagmus is a positive test.

Note
- Transient ischaemic attacks (TIA) do not cause syncope or pre-syncope.
- Isolated vertigo (i.e. no other associated neurological features) is always due to vestibular dysfunction.
- Consider hyperventilation as a cause of dizziness (reproduce symptoms by hyperventilating with the patient).
- Vasovagal syncope always occurs standing up; there is a clear precipitant (pain, fear, smell) and some presyncopal warning symptoms before the loss of consciousness.

Tests

If the patient is on insulin or sulphonylurea drugs (e.g. gliclazide), always test their blood sugar by glucometer (finger prick test).

Choice of tests will be guided by prior assessment. Increasingly this will be provided by specialist clinics and teams, but the basics should be known by all involved with older people.

If syncopal or presyncopal, postural blood pressure, ECG, echocardiography, and 24-h ECG can be useful. Other autonomic function tests (RR variation on ECG during deep breathing, Valsalva manoeuvre, or standing) may be useful to make the diagnosis of autonomic neuropathy. The diagnostic yield of echocardiography and 24-h ECG is low, and these tests should not be used indiscriminately in the absence of appropriate findings from the history or clinical examination.

A 24-h ECG recording can be difficult to interpret:
- It will often show multiple ventricular or supraventricular ectopic beats (of no significance), and even runs of such beats (of no particular diagnostic value).
- Paroxysmal AF requires that the rhythm be sustained for some minutes at least.
- There may episodes of bradycardia, particularly at night, which are only of importance if associated with second or third degree heart block, or if they are clearly symptomatic.
- Pauses less than 3 seconds are usually not significant.
- There may be false negatives—if there are no symptoms during the 24 h period, it is unlikely that a diagnostic rhythm will be captured. If the clinical features are sufficiently suspicious, you can go on to 48 or 72 h recordings, cardiomemo (a device that records during symptoms only), or an implantable loop recorder (like a pacemaker, which can be interrogated remotely electronically).

70° head up tilt testing is useful to investigate otherwise unexplained syncope, looking to diagnose carotid sinus hypersensitivity. However, this is lengthy (45–60 minutes), labour intensive to perform, and may give false positive results.

Blood count, erythrocyte sedimentation rate, renal and liver function, glucose and calcium are reasonable screening tests. Thyrotoxicosis and vitamin D status (PTH, 25-hydroxy vitamin D) can contribute to proximal muscle weakness. Vitamin B12 and folate deficiency can also cause neuropathy or other neurological symptoms.

CT or MRI scanning is only required when specifically indicated. Fits require neuroimaging. Otherwise a carefully conducted neurological examination, if normal, will generally exclude a structural neurological abnormality. Bony injury resulting from falls will require appropriate imaging.

Intervention

An identified precipitant or sufficient cause (e.g. arrhythmia or acute illness, 📖 Table 9.2) should be treated.

Careful medication review should be undertaken. Sedative, antipsychotic, and antidepressant drugs should be stopped unless:
- There is a clearly established appropriate diagnosis and indication.
- The continuing need for the drug has been reviewed and confirmed.
- There is clear evidence that starting the drug resulted in benefit. One way of establishing this is a stopping trial—Is there any evidence of deterioration on stopping the drug? (in which case it can be restarted).

One trial of drug minimization found that although they could successfully stop psychotropic drugs, and this reduced falls, participants usually restarted them within a year of stopping (📖 Box 9.2).

Box 9.2 Stopping psychotropic medication to reduce falls

- A cluster randomized trial was performed in 17 New Zealand general practices. 93 women and men aged over 65 years currently taking psychotropic medication were randomized to gradual withdrawal of psychotropic medication or continuing to take psychotropic medication.
- Relative risk for falls over 44 weeks of follow-up in the medication withdrawal group was 0.34 (95% CI 0.16–0.74).
- However, the majority of participants had restarted their psychotropic medication by the end of the study.

J Am Geriatr Soc 1999; **47**: 850–3.

Postural hypotension can be difficult to diagnose and manage:

- Drugs may be responsible, including antihypertensives, diuretics, anti-arrhythmics, antimuscarinic, and antipsychotics. Critically review the indication for all drugs. Sometimes they are prescribed for good reasons—such as to control heart failure or angina. Sometimes the indication is less clear, or less well justified. Diuretics are commonly prescribed for dependent oedema (ankle swelling due to immobility and inactivity). This is unsightly but harmless, unless it is so severe as to impede mobility. Ensure the patient sleeps in bed, not a chair, remains as mobile as possible and elevates the legs while sitting. Sacrifice antihypertensive drugs if they are causing problems. The danger from falling is both more immediate and greater than the danger from vascular risk.
- If this fails to resolve the problem, and the symptoms are sufficient to justify more than the advice to stand up slowly and wait a minute or so before walking off, elastic compression stockings can be suggested. These are uncomfortable and unpopular, especially in hot weather, but can be suggested and tried.
- After that try fludrocortisone, 100 mcg od increasing up to 300 mcg if required. There is no logic to this if the patient remains on diuretics (fludrocortisone retains sodium, diuretics offload it). Moreover, it often causes ankle swelling at doses above 100 mcg/d, and may cause hypokalaemia.
- Midodrine is an alpha agonist that can be effective, but it is unlicensed in the EU and only available on a named patient basis.

The second strand of management is to reduce the propensity to fall through the minimization of risk factors:

- The best-established intervention is physiotherapist-delivered strength and balance training. This has been refined in a series of trials, and is sometimes called the Otago exercise programme. Most falls prevention programmes are based around delivering this.
- Visual impairment should be diagnosed. Cataracts should be referred to an ophthalmologist; inadequate or out of date spectacles should be reviewed by an optometrist.
- Foot problems require chiropody.
- Environmental assessment and modification, usually by an occupational therapist, to reduce hazards, optimize equipment and appliances, and review lighting, are commonly employed in falls prevention programmes. Some of this is common sense and is required as part of a general rehabilitation assessment. In isolation, environmental assessment appears to be ineffective in preventing falls, but most would agree this should form part of a multi-faceted approach.

Vitamin D insufficiency (25-OH vitamin D <30 nmol/l) should be corrected. Some trials suggest that high dose calcium and vitamin D reduces the incidence of both falls and hip fracture by up to 50%. Subsequent trials have failed to replicate these findings, but in quite heterogeneous populations, so it is difficult to be sure that there is no benefit in some subgroups. There is sufficient evidence to justify treating all mobile care home residents (Box 9.3). However, for anyone at high risk of falling, 1 g of calcium and 800 units of vitamin D a day, in divided doses, seems sensible, and is more or less side effect free, so long as the person can take the fairly large tablets (or effervescent drink). Occasionally, someone with undiagnosed primary hyperparathyroidism will become hypercalcaemic. Those who have diagnosed osteoporosis will require it anyway as adjuvant therapy for bisphosphonates.

Box 9.3 Does calcium and vitamin D supplementation prevent falls or fractures?

- Vitamin D insufficiency is common amongst older people (up to 50% of at-risk populations). This, and a low calcium intake, contribute to secondary hyperparathyroidism and osteoporosis. Calcium and vitamin D supplements reduce hyperparathyroidism and increase bone mineral density.
- In a randomized controlled trial, 3270 ambulatory Swiss women, mean age 84 years, resident in residential homes (probably akin to British sheltered housing) were randomized to receive tricalcium phosphate (containing 1.2 g of elemental calcium) and 800 IU of vitamin D3 daily, or placebo.
- After 18 months follow-up, relative risk for treated women:
  - for hip fracture was 0.57 (p=0.04)
  - for total non-vertebral fractures was 0.68 (p=0.02).
- In the calcium-vitamin D3 group, after 18 months the mean serum parathyroid hormone concentration decreased 44% from baseline and the serum 25(OH) vitamin D concentration increased 162%.
- The bone density of the proximal femur increased 2.7% in the calcium-vitamin D group and decreased 4.6% in the placebo group.
- A Cochrane Library systematic review reported more equivocal results—vitamin D alone showed no statistically significant effect on:
  - Hip fracture RR 1.17 (95% CI 0.98–1.41) (seven trials, 18 668 participants).
  - Vertebral fracture RR 1.13 (95% CI 0.50–2.55) (four trials, 5698 participants).
  - Any new fracture RR 1.02 (95% CI 0.93–1.11) (eight trials, 18 935 participants).
- Vitamin D with calcium reduced:
  - Hip fractures RR 0.81 (95% CI 0.68–0.96) (seven trials, 10 376 participants).
  - Non-vertebral fractures RR 0.87 (95% CI 0.78–0.97) (seven trials, 10 376 participants), but not vertebral fractures.
- The effect appeared to be restricted to those living in institutional care.
- Analogues of vitamin D (calcitriol) showed no advantage over vitamin D itself.
- Hypercalcaemia was more common when vitamin D or its analogues were given compared with placebo or calcium (RR 2.38, 95% CI 1.52–3.71; 14 trials, 8035 participants). The risk was particularly high with calcitriol (RR 14.94, 95% CI 2.95–75.61; three trials, 742 participants). There was no significant increase in other side effects.

New Engl J Med 1992; **327**: 1637–42.
Cochrane Database of Systematic Reviews 2007; Issue 3.

It was hoped that hip protectors (a plastic or foam shield worn over the greater trochanter of the hip, sewn into pants) would give a good level of protection from hip fracture to people who continued to fall and who were happy to wear them. Trials suggested that fractures were rare amongst people who were actually wearing the hip protector at the time of the fall. Compliance was a problem—perhaps no more than 25% of people persisted. In the light of subsequent trials, efficacy is now in doubt (📖 Box 9.4).

Special problems in dementia

Multifactorial falls prevention intervention trials that have specifically targeted falls in dementia have been very disappointing (📖 Box 9.5).

This may mean that the main drivers for falls risk in dementia are different, or that the interventions require learning and behaviour change that are impossible in dementia. For example failure in anticipation, planning, judgement, and insight (self-appraisal of abilities) may be important, intrinsic to the condition, and unresponsive to advice and training. Failure to sustain attention (e.g. visual fixation, distractibility) might also be involved. A more 'neurological' explanation might involve weakness, apraxia, and impaired reaction times. The learning and repeated performance of exercises (which takes sustained commitment and hard work) may be impossible.

In positive terms, identifying and sorting out the 'quick wins' helps (cataracts, glasses, postural hypotension, sedative psychotropic and antidepressant drugs, foot problems, and inappropriate footwear). Improving mobility and sustaining fitness, strength, and stamina (mainly by walking practice) are also likely to help.

After that we are largely left with supervision and personal assistance during transfers and walking to avoid falls.

Box 9.4 Can hip protectors prevent hip fractures?

- An early trial suggested a substantial reduction in risk amongst nursing home residents randomized to wear hip protectors. Ten of the 28 wards in a Dutch nursing home were randomized to receive external hip protectors. 247 residents were given protectors and 418 residents had no protectors. A fall register was set up for two treatment wards (45 residents) and two control wards (76 residents).
- Relative risk of hip fractures among women and men in the intervention group was 0.44 (95% CI 0.21–0.94). There were 8 hip and 15 non-hip fractures in the hip protector group and 31 hip and 27 non-hip fractures in the control group.
- None of the eight residents in the intervention group who had a hip fracture was wearing the protector at the time. 154 falls were recorded. 20% of these falls produced direct impact on the hip. 25 falls caused direct impact to the hip at a time when hip protectors were not being worn, and six fractures resulted.
- Attempts to replicate this trial have been disappointing. For example a cluster randomized controlled trial randomized 127 nursing and residential homes in Northern Ireland. 40 homes were the intervention group (1366 beds) and 87 homes the control group (2751 beds).
- The intervention was to offer hip protectors (free of charge) to residents and to support implementation with a nurse facilitator to help staff in the homes to encourage their use.
- Adjusted rate ratio for falls over a 72-week period for the intervention group was 1.05 (95% CI 0.77–1.43). Mean fracture rate per 100 residents was 6.22 in the intervention homes (85 hip fractures) and 5.92 in the control homes (163 hip fractures). 37% of residents (508/1366) initially accepted hip protectors, but adherence fell to 20% (272/1366) by 72 weeks.
- A Cochrane systematic review identified 15 trials. In care homes, relative risk of fracture (RR) was 0.77 (95% CI 0.62–0.97). However, there was statistical heterogeneity amongst the trials (i.e. they varied one from another more than expected by chance, suggesting that the intervention was not the same everywhere, making the size of the pooled estimate of effect uncertain).
- In three individually randomized trials involving 5135 community dwelling participants, RR was 1.16 (95% CI 0.85–1.59) i.e. no reduction in hip fracture incidence from the provision of hip protectors. Compliance, particularly in the long term, was poor.
- Interpreting this evidence for clinical purposes is difficult. Randomized trials are designed to avoid giving positive results due to bias. They are less good at establishing that an intervention does not work, especially for subgroups (where power is rarely sufficient to exclude useful benefits). The main problem here could be non-compliance rather than ineffectiveness. This tells us little about whether they work in someone who is wearing them. For someone who is at very high risk, and who is comfortable with wearing hip protectors, and who can afford them (£100 for three pairs), they remain a reasonable option to discuss.

Lancet 1993; **341**: 11–3; *Age & Ageing* 2004; **33**: 582–8;
Cochrane Database of Systematic Reviews 2007; Issue 3.

Box 9.5 Randomized controlled trial to determine the effectiveness of multifactorial intervention after a fall in older patients with cognitive impairment attending an A&E department

- 274 cognitively impaired people aged 65 or over, with MMSE <24 (at presentation and remaining so 2 weeks later), who presented to two A&E departments after a fall, were randomized. Those with a clear medical cause for their fall, who were unable to walk or to communicate for reasons other than dementia, were excluded.
- 130 had assessment and multifactorial intervention. 144 received assessment followed by conventional care.
- Intervention comprised medical assessment (including drug review and assessment of vision and mood), extended cardiovascular assessment (ECG, lying and standing blood pressure, carotid sinus massage, and tilt test), physiotherapy assessment and supervised home-based strength, balance, and gait training, provision of appropriate aids and footwear, and occupational therapy for an environmental assessment.
- Mean age was 84 years and mean MMSE 13/30. 70% lived in care homes. 80% of the control patients fell in the follow-up year. Groups were well matched at baseline. 76% completed all the assessments. Compliance with interventions ranged from 50–85%.
- Relative risk of falling over in the follow-up year was 0.92 (95% CI 0.81–1.05). None of various secondary outcomes (fall rate, injury, or hospital admission) showed significant differences between groups.
- Gait score, environmental risk score, extent of postural drop in blood pressure, and prevalence of cardio-inhibitory carotid sinus syndrome all improved in the intervention group, but no more than could have been explained by chance.
- The study concluded that multifactorial intervention was not effective in preventing falls in older people with cognitive impairment presenting to the A&E department after a fall.
- The study was relatively small, with minor baseline imbalance, and only moderate compliance. The statistical analysis was very conservative, and the confidence intervals could not exclude a moderate sized benefit, so, whilst disappointing, the study does not exclude a beneficial effect of intervention. Applicability to fitter community-dwelling older people is uncertain.

BMJ 2003; **326**: 73–9

Hip fracture

A hip fracture results from an interplay of three things:
- Trauma, usually a fall (1% of hip fractures are said to be spontaneous).
- Sufficient impact (and 'correct' geometry) to break the bone.
- Bone that is weak enough to break, usually due to osteoporosis.

Hip fracture, stroke and dementia, form the 'big three' disabling conditions of extreme old age. Its incidence increases exponentially with age. A third of victims are dead within a year of a hip fracture.

Initial management is surgical. The fracture should be operatively fixed within 24 h unless a comorbid medical condition makes delay desirable whilst medical stabilization occurs. Internal fixation provides excellent pain relief, and is therefore indicated even in the very frail and terminally ill.

Depending on the type of fracture the patient can be mobilized the day following surgery (hemiarthroplasty for transcervical fracture) or within 3 days (dynamic hip screws for intertrochanteric fracture—these tend to be more painful post-operatively). Complex or comminuted fractures may require prolonged (6–8 weeks) immobilization after operation to allow stable bone healing.

Rehabilitation largely focuses on restoring walking, initially with the support of a pulpit or gutter frame. The main approach is progressive supervised practice to build strength, balance, stamina, cardio-respiratory fitness, and confidence. Most patients will achieve functional mobility within a fortnight, but walking should continue to improve for several months afterwards. This can be managed mostly by home rehabilitation or other intermediate care. Frailer patients or those with severe comorbidities may require prolonged in-patient rehabilitation (up to several months). Adequate pain control is important to facilitate this.

Patients with dementia fare variably, but overall less well than the cognitively intact. Some walk again quickly, others fail to respond to physiotherapy instruction or lose confidence, whereupon deconditioning rapidly compounds the problem. Good liaison with psychiatric services or an interested geriatrician reduces mortality and length of hospital stay after hip fracture.

Medical comorbidity and complications are very common. Frequently acute or acute on chronic medical problems contribute to the initial fall, and patients arrive at hospital unfit for surgery, requiring initial medical and anaesthetic intervention. Delirium, chest and other infections, dehydration or electrolyte disturbance, cardiac failure, and venous thromboembolism all frequently arise, making early joint management with a geriatrician an important aspect of management. Patients are often catheterized at some stage, risking infection and inhibiting mobility. This should be removed as soon as is feasible.

Management should include:
- Identifying why the patient fell and whether intervention is required to prevent further falls.
- Identifying and optimizing comorbidities, and rationalizing medications.
- Management of osteoporosis—it is safe to assume that all older people with a hip fracture are osteoporotic. Most should be given high dose calcium and vitamin D, and a weekly bisphosphonate, subject to medicines management being feasible.

Immobility

Immobility describes an 'activity limitation' or 'disability'. As such it is often the end result of multiple pathologies and other factors, although a single sufficient cause may be identifiable.

A common crisis is when someone has 'gone off their legs' due to an acute or acute on chronic illness. Immobility is another of the 'geriatric giants', the non-specific presentations of acute disease. It also results from chronic illness, including musculo-skeletal, neurological, cardio-respiratory, and dementia.

An important additional feature is the role of 'deconditioning': the loss of muscular strength and stamina, and cardio-respiratory fitness, following a period of illness, immobility, or under-activity. The good news is that this is reversible with sustained and progressive exercise, and, along with restoration of confidence, probably accounts for a large part of what is achieved in general geriatric rehabilitation.

The medical model calls for assessment and identification of causes, intervention to reverse the treatable causes and palliate outstanding symptoms, and rehabilitation to improve motor function and other functional abilities.

Gross mobility can be quantified at a series of levels (🔲 Box 9.6). Further qualification can be in terms of:
• Human help (number of persons, hands on or supervision).
• Aids required (wheelchair, pulpit frame, gutter frame, wheeled Zimmer frame, three-wheeled delta frame, crutches, sticks).
• Degree of difficulty experienced.
• Distance or speed achieved.

A report may for example describe someone as being able to walk 10 m with a Zimmer frame and the supervision of one person.

Causes of immobility

Assessment will identify the symptoms and signs (impairments) leading to the problem (Table 9.3). Impairments must be explained by diagnoses. This requires proper history taking and thorough examination of the neurological and musculo-skeletal systems, heart, and chest. Reports from nurses and therapists provide useful insight into problems.

Always consider an acute medical illness (infection, metabolic disturbance, new stroke, drug side effect) when mobility declines suddenly. Immobility may not be 'curable' but at a minimum do not miss a treatable cause. Consider if part, at least, of a progressive decline might be due to deconditioning, which is eminently reversible. After an acute illness, the ambition should always be a return to pre-morbid mobility, regardless of cognitive ability.

Box 9.6 Describing and quantifying mobility

- Head control.
- Rolling in bed.
- Static sitting balance.
- Dynamic sitting balance.
- Bed to chair transfer.
- Rising from sitting to standing.
- Sustained standing.
- Stepping round to transfer.
- Walking on the flat indoors.
- Stair climbing.
- Walking outdoors.

Table 9.3 Causes of immobility

System	Problem	Intervention
Musculo-skeletal	Arthritis, especially knees, hips, back	Analgesia, exercise, intra-articular steroid injection, arthroplasty
	Covert fractures (pelvis, hip, tibeal plateau)	X-ray, analgesia, fixation, physiotherapy
	Limb loss	Prosthesis, wheelchair
	Foot deformities (toenails, ulcers, hallux valgus)	Chiropody, wound care, surgery
	Myopathy (vitamin D, thyroid, steroid, myositis)	Diagnosis, routine calcium and vitamin D supplementation, steroid reduction or avoidance
Neurological	Hemiparesis (usually stroke)	Diagnosis, rehabilitation
	Paraparesis (including spinal cord compression, cervical myelopathy)	Diagnosis, possibly surgery, rehabilitation
	Parkinson's disease	Remove drug causes, drug treatment, rehabilitation
	Peripheral neuropathy	Diagnosis, foot care, walking aids
Vision	Blindness	Diagnosis, refraction, cataract surgery, low vision aids, supervision
	Hemianopia and inattention	Training in compensation, supervision
Cardiovascular	Heart failure (breathlessness, oedema)	Diagnose and treat cause (muscle disease, valve, rhythm), diuretics, ACE inhibitor, beta blocker, secondary prevention
	Chest pain	Diagnose, antianginal drugs, angiography and revascularization, secondary prevention
	Postural hypotension	Reduce culprit drugs, hosiery, fludrocortisone
	Intermittent claudication	Walking, secondary prevention, angiography and revascularization
Respiratory	Breathlessness (COPD, pulmonary embolism, fibrosis, effusion, pneumonia, cancer)	Diagnosis, stop smoking, bronchodilators or other therapy as indicated

Table 9.3 Causes of immobility

System	Problem	Intervention
Skin	Leg or foot ulcers	Remove trauma (including 4 layer compression bandaging for venous, revascularization for arterial, orthotic shoes for neuropathic feet), treat infection, debride, dress to keep moist, treat anaemia, good diet (protein, zinc, vitamin C)
	Oedema (dependency, heart failure, hypoalbumenaemia, venous or lymphatic obstruction)	Diagnose. Low doses of diuretics (up to 40 mg furosemide) may help, but usually at the cost of intravascular depletion, which can cause problems.
Psychological	Anxiety, loss of confidence	Supervised practice, reassurance
	Depression with psychomotor retardation	Treat. Supervised practice, reassurance
	Dementia (apraxia, executive failure)	Supervised practice

Dementia impacts on the ability to engage with complex instructions and learn new ways of performing motor tasks. Therapists refer to the degree of 'carry over'—the ability to remember from one session to another, so that each session can build on what was achieved in the last and activity can progress to more difficult levels. This should be judged on a case-by-case basis. Rehabilitation therapists not experienced in working with people with dementia should beware of making gloomy assumptions about prognosis.

Sometimes a 'functional approach' is required—the finer points of ideal therapy practice are abandoned to concentrate on repeated performance of practical tasks (such as walking or dressing). This often works, because many day to day activities, including walking, are well-engrained in the long-term (implicit) memory (☐ Box 6.3) and can be accessed with sufficient persistence and practice. Rehabilitation may take longer, and the context may be one of longer-term progressive decline. What is required, realistic, and achievable should be negotiated as part of goal setting.

Clearly more major interventions (such as joint replacement) should be considered very carefully, using the usual decision-making process (☐ Chapter 12). There may be real benefits to be gained, but the possibility of a long period of debility without ultimate benefit has to be considered if rehabilitation cannot be successfully achieved.

Rehabilitation is hard work. It is not a process of passive receiving; rather it requires prolonged active participation. Issues of 'motivation' and 'engagement' become frustrating for therapy staff and nurses. Foresight, planning, and decision-making may be affected, especially in frontal type dementia. The patient may find therapy effortful or unpleasant, and if they forget why they are doing it, or fail to realize that a stated goal (like going home) depends on achieving intermediate tasks (like walking), they may decline to take part. Gentle persuasion and encouragement helps, and on occasions a more assertive approach is needed (almost 'bullying'). A growing tendency to disengage when superficially taken 'consent' is not gained is probably not in most demented patients' best interests. If engagement really is impossible, then further attempts are futile, a halt should be called, and alternative plans made.

Sometimes in advanced dementia the onset of immobility can be a welcome development, as it reduces problems with agitation and aggression.

Urinary tract infection (UTI)

These are common but complex, and the diagnosis is hopelessly overused as an explanation for acute deteriorations in confused older people, often without any justification.

UTI may be:
• Symptomatic or asymptomatic. Typical symptoms are a burning dysuria, sometimes described as like passing broken glass, and increased urinary frequency and urgency (in effect, the inflamed bladder becomes unstable). 30% of elderly women have asymptomatic bacturia. In the context of acute illness these are impossible to define (what is the symptom?) and treatment is inevitable. UTI is relatively rare in men (unless catheterized or with incomplete bladder emptying)—never assume it unless there is at least some confirmatory evidence.
• Present atypically—with delirium, falls, or agitation.
• Recurrent. Risk factors include being catheterized, a post-menopausal woman, or having a urinary residual.

Diagnosis
• Consider if there are systemic features, such as delirium, incontinence, pyrexia, neutrophilia, or raised inflammatory markers (e.g. C-reactive protein).
• Screen with a dipstick. If negative for leucocyte esterase and nitrites, UTI is unlikely. Otherwise send for culture (i.e. you can exclude UTI with a dipstick test, but not confirm it).
• Culture and sensitivity. If a delay is likely before processing use boric acid preservative in the bottle (often with a red top for the specimen bottle).
• Identify a predisposition or cause. Catheters are obvious. If recurrent, check post-void residual urinary volume (by ultrasound); consider atrophic urethritis and imaging the upper urinary tracts (by ultrasound) for stones, obstruction, or scarring.

Treatment
• Treat the infection, and the predisposition.
• Three days of antibiotics are sufficient for uncomplicated infections in most women (i.e. not catheterized or other structural abnormality, not pyelonephritis). Seven days for men.
• Review the need for a urethral catheter. If long-term catheterization is inevitable, colonization infections are inevitable. Treat them as they occur if they are causing problems.
• If symptoms are suggestive but cultures negative this suggests a urethral syndrome—caused by oestrogen deficiency (atrophic urethritis) or infection (consider chlamydia or other sexually transmitted infections). Give estradiol (e.g. Vagifem®) to women, take a swab, and consider an empirical 2-week course of a tetracycline (doxycline 100 mg od for 14 days). Consider other causes of irritation (lichen sclerosus, irritants such as soap or antiseptics).

Urinary incontinence

Urinary incontinence

Definition

Urinary incontinence is 'the complaint of any involuntary leakage of urine'. An older qualification that the leakage should cause a social or hygienic problem was dropped as being ambiguous, not least because of the problem of insight in dementia, raising the question 'In whose opinion?' For our purposes an even wider definition may be useful: 'The failure to pass urine or faeces in a socially acceptable place.'

Continence is defined by social and cultural norms. The driver by the roadside and the drunken rugby player in the sink are not generally thought incontinent. 'Socially acceptable' is modified by ill health. The range of places may extend to urinals, commodes, or chemical toilets in the bedroom or living room.

Bladder muscle function may be affected in any neurological disease:

- Dementia is associated with detrusor hyper-reflexia (an unstable bladder, which contracts before it is full and when the patient does not want it to due to a failure of inhibition of detrusor contractions).
- Frontal lobe lesions sometimes result in an extreme form of this—urinary precipitancy, where there is no warning at all.

The problem may also be due to comorbid pathology:

- 10% of the general population and 20% of people over 70 have detrusor instability.
- Causes of detrusor instability also include idiopathic primary detrusor instability, prostatic enlargement, oestrogen deficiency, stones, or bladder cancer.
- Incomplete bladder emptying is most often due to prostate disease, faecal impaction, or antimuscarinic drugs, but a proportion have idiopathic detrusor underactivity, including some women.
- Incontinence of urine is common in acute medical illness and delirium—this so-called 'transient' incontinence accounts for 50% of incontinence in acute hospitals and 30% in the community. It resolves with treatment of the acute illness.

Patients may not have bladder or bowel dysfunction but toileting or orientation difficulty (so-called 'functional incontinence'). A range of problems includes:

- Anticipating the need to void or open bowels.
- Recognition when need is imminent.
- Finding and recognizing the toilet (or other acceptable place), especially in unfamiliar surroundings.
- Getting there, especially if mobility is impaired, if some form of (covert) restraint is in place, or if the need is urgent.
- Summoning help if it is required.
- Manipulating clothing (including possibly an incontinence pad).
- Inhibitions about using unfamiliar toilets (especially women).
- Bottom wiping afterwards.

Relevant disorders may therefore include: judgement and planning; awareness; depression; disorientation in place; agnosia; ability to stand; walking speed; lethargy, pain, or breathlessness; postural stability; negotiating restrictive chairs, tables, bed rails, doors, or stairs; asking for and waiting for help; manual dexterity and dressing apraxia; embarrassment, confidence, fear, or habit; detrusor instability or disinhibited colonic reflex.

Someone voiding in the sink or opening their bowels into a waste paper basket may have good bladder or bowel control, and may have been trying desperately to remain continent, but may simply have failed to find an 'acceptable place'. The most appropriate response may be a compliment for damage limitation (better than wetting the bed or soiling clothes), rather than admonition or the application of pads.

Success in improving continence may be short lived as the disease progresses.

Consequences

Disruption in bladder and bowel function can result in:
- Distress and embarrassment for the patient.
- Change in relationships with carers.
- Inability of carers to cope with washing, changing, and handling urine and faeces or soiled clothes.
- Carers feeling it is done 'on purpose'.
- Risk of abuse from care workers through fatigue, anger, or punishment (as a misplaced crude psychological approach).
- Request for care home placement.

Assessment and diagnosis

An individual approach is required, and assessment is the key to this. This may take some time to complete and must be reviewed as the patient's condition changes. It is essential to work with family or paid carers to gather information. Include:
- Medical and bladder history.
- Past life history, particularly relating to bladder and bowel rituals, practices.
- Bladder and bowel symptoms.
- Post void residual volume measurement (preferably by ultrasound scanner, or by residual catheterization if ultrasound is unavailable).
- Bladder diary for 3 days (or a toileting chart where there is 24 h care).
- If possible complete a 3 day frequency-volume chart. This will give an idea of functional bladder capacity (which is low in instability, often less than 200 ml), total urine output, and the day-night split of output. If the patient is incontinent into pads, these can be weighed to estimate voided volume. Pads can be tied into plastic bags for later weighing if the patient is at home.
- Use Newcastle urine collector if there is difficulty obtaining a urine specimen.
- Urinalysis to include leucocytes, nitrites, protein, blood, and glucose.
- Send urine for culture if not negative for leucocytes and nitrites.
- If there is haematuria this may require investigation. The risk of stones or renal or bladder cancer is low if there is isolated microscopic haematuria, but most guidelines suggest investigating anyway if microscopic haematuria persists.

Management

- If there is infection, treat it.
- Ensure a reasonable fluid intake—aim for 2 litres a day plus what comes in food. Avoid caffeine, although rapid caffeine withdrawal symptoms can be unpleasant. Concentrated urine and caffeine both irritate the bladder.
- Review timing of fluid intake, especially if there are night time problems. Large volumes of beer or bedtime drinks will inevitably lead to the need to void overnight.
- Review diabetic control.
- Review the need for culprit drugs, especially furosemide. It may be possible to reduce the dose (down to as little as 20 mg), split the dose, or use a slower onset, longer acting alternative such as torasemide.
- Add an antimuscarinic if there is urgency, or functional bladder capacity is low, and the residual volume is less than 100 ml. The newer bladder-selective drugs provide the best balance between efficacy and side effects (mainly dry mouth and heartburn). However, these drugs are prone to cause delirium and cognitive function can be made worse by antimuscarinic drugs. Newer drugs (e.g. trospium 20 mg bd) cross the blood-brain barrier least, and therefore are the drugs of choice in dementia. None of the antimuscarinic drugs is dramatically effective. In trials, cystometric bladder capacity increased from about 200 ml to 250 ml (normal capacity 400–600 ml, a little lower in an older person).
- Cholinesterase inhibitors used as anti-dementia drugs can make incontinence worse; in such cases trospium is usually well-tolerated and helpful.
- Always review drug treatment for effectiveness. Antimuscarinic drugs will rarely solve a urinary problem completely, but may help. The risk is abandoning a useful treatment when a residual problem remains. A repeat frequency volume chart is the best way of determining this, but a simple tick-chart may suffice. Also review for side effects.
- Try prompted voiding every 2–3 hours.
- Vaginal oestrogens sometimes relieve urgency and can be a helpful adjunct (creams are messy—use estradiol vaginal tablets 'Vagifem®').
- Consider the possibility of genuine stress incontinence (leakage on raising abdominal pressure without detrusor contractions). The first line treatment is pelvic floor re-education, but this requires considerable technique (nurses or physiotherapists should teach it using vaginal examination to be effective), co-operation, and persistence (3–5 times a day for 3 months) and will be beyond many with dementia. Pelvic floor contraction helps inhibit unstable detrusor contractions, so there is some benefit from pelvic floor exercises regardless of diagnosis. There may also be an associated cystocoele that needs diagnosing and appropriate management.
- If there is retention, try a Queens Square Bladder Stimulator (a vibrating massaging device), intermittent catheterization, or an alpha blocker. Doxazosin 1 mg increasing to 4 mg od (needs titrating up to avoid postural hypotension), or doxazosin MR 4 mg od, can be co-indicated as antihypertensives. Tamsulosin MR 400 mcg od is uroselective and has less effect on blood pressure.

- If unsuccessful, optimize containment:
  - For men try a sheath catheter (penile size should not matter).
  - Otherwise try pads. These have a capacity up to 1100 ml, but if saturated are heavy (1100 g).
  - Indwelling catheters are a last resort. They always get infected, block, or bypass due to bladder spasm. An antimuscarinic drug may be needed to reduce spasm. Do not shrink from a 'trial of catheter' if that is what the duly-informed patient wants, and it is the only way to get someone home. The usually well-justified reluctance to use catheters can be taken too far.
  - Consider a suprapubic catheter if intended as a long-term solution—they are more comfortable and less prone to infection.

Other urinary symptoms

Other urinary symptoms can be equally troublesome, in particular urgency and nocturia. The need for multiple transfers onto the commode or trips to the toilet at night is a major falls risk and can place considerable strain on a spouse or cohabiting carer.

- Urgency almost always means detrusor instability, but can sometimes indicate incomplete bladder emptying. Do a bladder scan and then try an antimuscarinic drug, and review.
- Nocturia can indicate:
  - Unstable bladder—should be detectable from frequent low volume voids on the frequency-volume chart.
  - Insomnia—ask about pain, anxiety, and depression. Insomnia increases both urine output (there is no sleep-associated ADH surge) and awareness of a filling bladder.
  - Incomplete bladder emptying—this will need relieving medically (alpha blockers), surgically (TURP), or with a catheter (intermittent if possible).
  - Nocturnal polyuria—night time (8 h, whilst asleep) output should be less than one-third of total output. Normal urine output rate is 70–100 ml/h depending on fluid intake. The normal young adult circadian rhythm in ADH-vasopressin secretion reduces this to 35 ml/h during sleep. Causes of nocturnal polyuria include diabetes, alcohol consumption, oedema, lithium therapy, heart failure, hypercalcaemia, and, most commonly, age-related nocturnal polyuria. If the latter, this is a combined loss of diurnal variation in vasopressin secretion and partial renal unresponsiveness to it (i.e. partial cranial and partial nephrogenic diabetes insipidus). Try giving chlortalidone 100 mg bd, decreasing to 50 mg od after a month (this has a paradoxical anti-diuretic action by sensitizing renal tubules to ADH). It often cuts night time output by about a half. Furosemide 40 mg in the morning sometimes helps, but causes urinary problems of

its own. Desmopressin 200–400 mcg given 6 nights in 7 sometimes works, but is often disappointing in practice. Moreover, in the UK it is not licensed for use in people over 65, who are more prone to hyponatraemia and who are often hypertensive. Tricyclic antidepressants (e.g. dosulepin 50–75 mg at night) can increase ADH secretion and are sedative and bladder stabilizing, but are also antimuscarinic so may worsen cognition. Lithium-associated polyuria responds to amiloride 5–10 mg od, but watch for electrolyte disturbance and lithium toxicity (check levels after a week).

Constipation

- Constipation is the infrequent or difficult passage of faeces, excessive straining in an attempt to pass stool, or the feeling of incomplete emptying after bowel opening.
- Normal bowel function is variable—'three times a day to once every three days.' Strictly, many older people, and even more with dementia, are constipated. Indeed, most Western non-vegetarians have harder stools than we were designed for. 40% of elderly people admitted to medical wards have rectal loading with hard faeces.
- Faecal impaction implies the presence of a mass of hard stool in the rectum and descending colon that cannot be passed spontaneously. In severe cases this may lead on to bowel obstruction, with abdominal discomfort, distension, and vomiting.
- Use the Bristol stool scale to define consistency (see Box 9.7). Types 1–2 are undesirably hard, 3–5 normal, 6–7 diarrhoea.

Box 9.7 The Bristol stool scale

Type 1: Separate hard lumps, like nuts (hard to pass).
Type 2: Sausage-shaped but lumpy.
Type 3: Like a sausage but with cracks on its surface.
Type 4: Like a sausage or snake, smooth and soft.
Type 5: Soft blobs with clear-cut edges (easily passed).
Type 6: Fluffy pieces with ragged edges, a mushy stool.
Type 7: Watery, no solid pieces, entirely liquid.

Causes of constipation include immobility, poor dietary fibre (fruit and vegetable) intake, poor fluid intake, drugs (opiates, antimuscarinic, calcium channel blockers, iron), metabolic causes (hypothyroidism, hypercalcaemia), spinal cord disease, autonomic dysfunction, and obstructing colonic lesions (which more often cause diarrhoea).

- Constipation *per se* is unlikely to be a cause of confusion, but it may cause agitation.
- Treatment of constipation is with laxatives or enemas. Avoid constipating drugs and ensure adequate fluid intake. A footstool may help improve body position for defecation (plastic stools designed to help little boys stand at the toilet are ideal). Encourage mobility and adequate dietary fibre.
- Laxatives divide between stool softeners and stimulants. Combining the two is logical.
- Stimulants include senna (15–30 mg/d), bisacodyl (can cause colic) and danthron (in the UK only licensed for terminal disease, which in context is unlikely to be an issue, but it may also cause a burn-like skin rash). Long-term (20 years plus) use of stimulants can cause colonic immotility and intractable constipation. However, stimulant laxatives should always be co-prescribed (or at least considered) with opiate analgesics.
- Softeners include docusate sodium (200 mg bd), which is the drug of choice in this situation, ispaghula husk (e.g. Fybogel®), and macrogols (e.g. Movicol®). Lactulose is relatively ineffective. Ispaghula husk is made up as a 200 ml drink, which often sets in the glass and can be difficult to take. Macrogols are a useful add-in when alternatives fail, and can be easily titrated up according to response (including a regimen licensed for impaction). Magnesium sulfate can be used in a similar way, as can small doses of sodium picosulfate (half a sachet at a time).
- Enemas and suppositories are disliked by patients (micro-enemas somewhat less so) but may be necessary. They can either be stimulants (Microlax®, glycerine suppository) or softeners (arachis oil).
- Rarely, manual disimpaction is required.

Faecal incontinence

- This is very common, becoming more prevalent as dementia severity worsens. It affects the majority of nursing home residents with dementia, and is almost universal in end-stage disease.
- Persisting and uncontrolled faecal incontinence is a major barrier to remaining at home.
- Seek a cause (Box 9.8) but don't expect this to be easy.
- Many patients are constipated. The rectum is a mucus-producing organ, and a hard faecal mass stimulates its production, which then leaks out as 'spurious diarrhoea'. A rectal examination (and in hospital often an abdominal X-ray) is required.
- A disinhibited colon due to dementia is unlikely to recover. Try to anticipate bowel opening (keep a bowel chart). It may occur regularly at a particular time of day, e.g. after getting up or after a meal.
- If remaining at home, or a discharge home, depends on continence, initiate a bowel regime (loperamide 2–16 mg/d to induce constipation, then arrange enemas 2–3 times a week for a controlled bowel evacuation). Patients find this unpleasant. Otherwise, ensure adequate containment (pads), and that they are changed quickly if soiled.
- Incontinence due to diarrhoea needs investigation in its own right.
- Be aware of drug-induced diarrhoea (laxatives, antibiotics, iron, proton pump inhibitors, and metformin).

Box 9.8 Causes of faecal incontinence

- Constipation with overflow incontinence.
- Disinhibited 'neurogenic' colon.
- Diarrhoea.
- Laxatives or other drugs.
- Diminished level of consciousness or unawareness.
- Immobility.
- Anorectal sphincter damage.

Pain

Pain is a symptom that may indicate disease and therefore requires diagnosis. Removal of unpleasant symptoms is also a good thing in its own right. Towards the end of life, relief of pain and other distress may be the overriding objective. Otherwise, the problem is in achieving a balance between effectiveness, side effects, and the burden of tablet taking.

However, diagnosis is difficult. People with moderate or advanced dementia have great difficulty articulating a cause for their distress. They may be unable to describe the pain, or lack the ability for abstract thought. Ideas of improvement or deterioration are difficult as dementia compromises perception of passage of time.

Any change in behaviour, such as aggression, shouting, or refusing to eat, may be caused by pain. It is often impossible to distinguish between distress of different causes; similar symptoms may be produced by a fracture or by being in a strange and threatening place. For known painful conditions, people with dementia are offered less in the way of analgesia than people who can talk about their pain.

Pain usually indicates tissue damage, but its perception is heavily coloured by mood or other psychological processes. Both must be assessed.

Where possible, localize and characterize pain. Describe:
- Number of different pains.
- Duration, progression, variation.
- Site and radiation.
- Type of pain, using descriptive terms.
- Precipitating and relieving factors.
- Treatments already tried.
- Effect on sleep.
- Non-verbal cues to pain (wincing, withdrawal).
- Impact on activities.
- Bothersomeness.
- Expectations.

Diagnose the pain. Common sources are:
- Arthritis and degenerative back disease, including osteoarthritis, rheumatoid disease, gout, and pseudogout.
- Other musculo-skeletal pain, including fractures, muscular, ligament, and tendon pain.
- Ischaemic pain, including angina, intermittent claudication, and ischaemic ulcers.
- Neuropathic pain (typically burning or shooting, with allodynia, the unpleasant perception of normal stimuli, and usually reduced sensation), radicular pain, and central pain (e.g. post stroke).
- Cancer pain, including visceral, serosal, and bony pain.
- Headache, including tension headache, migraine, temporal arteritis, and raised intra-cranial pressure.

Pain that is ill-defined, all over the body, unvarying, and very long-standing is more likely to represent depression than tissue damage, especially in cultures where psychological symptoms are poorly accepted.

In dementia we are more reliant on descriptions of the here and now. Moreover, at times repeated complaints of pain may represent repetitiveness rather than therapeutic failure.

Address the underlying cause if possible.

Setting realistic and achievable objectives is important. Complete abolition of pain will often not be possible, so minimize its impact without causing new problems. Clearly, relieving distressing pain towards the end of life is a high priority, and adverse effects (e.g. drowsiness or worse cognition) may be acceptable trade-offs.

The foundation of all analgesic regimens is *regular* paracetamol (1 g qds). It is virtually side effect free, and whilst only moderately strong, may take the edge off pain sufficiently to make it bearable. It can be taken in the long term and should be continued even when stronger analgesics are added in.

All other analgesics carry a burden of adverse effects. Weak opioids (codeine, dihydrocodeine) are very prone to cause delirium, constipation, and nausea, and in general should be avoided in people with cognitive impairment. Tramadol (50–100 mg qds) may be better tolerated, but can also cause delirium and constipation, and opinions about its usefulness are divided.

Stronger opiates share these side effects, but can be very useful in context, especially fracture pain, cancer pain, and terminal care. Morphine can be started at a very low dose and titrated up as required. There are both standard and sustained-release formulations. Oxycodone is a good alternative if there are problems—some people are more prone to side effects from particular opiates in an apparently idiosyncratic way.

Some newer formulations and delivery routes (e.g. low dose transdermal buprenorphine or fentanyl) can be tried with care. All generally require co-prescription of a stimulant laxative (senna, danthron), and may initially require an antiemetic (cyclizine). Low dose haloperidol (1–2 mg/d) is a useful antiemetic that has a synergistic analgesic effect as well as its anxiolytic properties.

Non-steroidal anti-inflammatory drugs are useful at times, but risk dyspepsia, peptic ulceration, renal dysfunction, and fluid retention (e.g. ibuprofen 400 mg tds, naproxen 250–500 mg bd, or diclofenac 50 mg tds). Co-prescribe a proton pump inhibitor (e.g. lansoprazole 30 mg od) unless a Cox-2 selective inhibitor (e.g. celecoxib) is used. Overall, however, these are no safer than older non-selective drugs. They are useful for inflammatory pain (gout, pleurisy) and pain from bony metastases.

Neuropathic pain is difficult to diagnose (or exclude). It may respond to pregabalin (50–100 mg tds) or gabapentin (although the latter is difficult and slow to titrate up). Side effects are a potential problem (especially drowsiness), but the alternative (amitriptyline) is worse.

Consider non-analgesic approaches (acupuncture, TENS). Antidepressants (SSRIs or TCAs) can be useful adjuvants.

Don't forget specialist pain services in selected difficult cases, especially if you know what you are after (e.g. a nerve block, epidural, or palliative radiotherapy for bony metastases). Otherwise a clinic practitioner who does not know the patient and is unused to managing dementia may struggle to make a meaningful assessment.

Remember to review analgesic prescriptions regularly, and stop stronger drugs if a transient cause of pain has passed.

Parkinsonism

Parkinsonism is the combination of:
- Increased tone, usually with cogwheel pattern.
- Bradykinesia.
- Tremor.
- Loss of postural reflexes.

Parkinsonism and cognitive impairment is a common and difficult combination, arising in several ways:
- Dementia with Lewy bodies—Parkinsonism is part of the syndrome.
- Dementia in pre-existing idiopathic Parkinson's disease.
- Delirium caused by antiparkinsonian drugs (especially antimuscarinic and dopamine agonists).
- Cerebrovascular disease with cognitive impairment and Parkinsonism.
- Drug-induced Parkinsonism (phenothiazines, remembering that metoclopramide and prochlorperazine are dopamine antagonists; occasionally selective serotonin reuptake inhibitors).

Particular problems occur with gait, falls, speech, posture, and sometimes swallowing or constipation. Treatment of idiopathic Parkinson's disease, in its early stages at least, is successful with one or both of dopamine agonists (such as ropinirole) and/or levodopa/dopa decarboxylase inhibitor combinations. However, people with dementia (especially DLB, 📖 Chapter 1) are likely to suffer psychotic side effects with dopamine agonists, and if treatment is tried it is best to go straight to levodopa.

Unfortunately, as the disease progresses, treatment with levodopa becomes less successful, with doses tending to wear off before the next one is due, the development of dose-related dyskinesias (writhing movements) as the dose of levodopa is increased to compensate, and unpredictable freezing episodes. These effects can develop as early as a year after starting treatment; on average patients get 7 years of good response to levodopa.

In response to this, several strategies have emerged. In younger patients levodopa is avoided for as long as possible by initial use of dopamine agonists. However, both these and antimuscarinic drugs (e.g. trihexyphenidyl) previously used in this role are best avoided in dementia. Fluctuations are reduced by using sustained release preparations (e.g. co-careldopa MR) or by adding one or other of a monoamine oxidase type B inhibitor (selegiline) or a catechol-O-methyl transferase inhibitor (entacapone). Parenteral apomorphine can be added for freezing episodes (after pre-treating for a week with domperidone).

Drug treatment of all Parkinsonian syndromes other than idiopathic Parkinson's disease is disappointing, although 25% of people with DLB achieve motor benefit with levodopa. Often a treatment trial (or its converse, a stopping trial) is required to establish if there is an effect or not. Make a baseline assessment such as a timed walk or get up and go test. Then start a low dose (e.g. co-beneldopa 12.5/50 tds) for a week and reassess. Then double the dose and repeat the assessment after a further week. Abandon drug therapy if there is no clear benefit.

'Clinical judgement'

Dementia does not make the management of 'physical problems' easy, but nor does it excuse neglect of them.

Real difficulties must be acknowledged with tolerating investigations, medicines management, adverse drug effects, decision-making and consent, and engagement in rehabilitation therapies. But we must still try. Therapeutic nihilism is unjustified. However, diagnostic obsession and defensive medicine are not excusable either.

The decision-making framework can help us here (📖 Chapter 12). Consider explicitly benefits, burdens, autonomy or best interests, and avoiding discrimination. This implies a greater need for communication and discussion with patients and their carers than usual, and the agreement of achievable goals.

Patients and their carers expect information about available options, but above all they want an opinion about the best way forward. Spell out the explicit risks, but also be realistic about the chances of success or likely useful intervention. For example, an asymptomatic iron deficiency anaemia is discovered. Stomach or bowel cancer could be the cause, but gastro-intestinal tract investigation is unpleasant. If cancer were diagnosed would it be potentially operable? Would the patient want or be fit for potentially curative surgery if it were? Don't presuppose the answers, but do ask the questions.

Waiting and seeing can be equally good management.

Summary

1. Multiple pathology implies multiple opportunities to intervene. But polypharmacy, with uncertain compliance and risk of side effects, is a problem. Stopping and starting drugs is one of the easiest things doctors do. Take clinical therapeutics seriously and get it right.

2. The assessment and prevention of falling is a major geriatric sub-specialty, with well-defined expertise and dedicated services. People with dementia fall more often than the cognitively intact, but fare less well in prevention programmes.

3. Hip fracture is often a tragedy, but some people with dementia rehabilitate well, if slowly. Assess the cause of the fall, need for osteoporosis treatment, and burden of comorbidity.

4. Urinary incontinence has many causes, but fairly few clinical manifestations (overactive bladder or retention). Incontinence is part of the syndrome of delirium and may appear during any acute illness. Often incontinence in dementia is intractable, but not always. Test for infection and incomplete bladder emptying. Regular prompted voiding may control the problem. If not, arrange adequate containment.

5. Faecal incontinence and constipation are common and distressing. Both require diagnosis and explanation. Constipation is easy to treat, but don't miss an underlying cause. Incontinence may be due to constipation or diarrhoea, which may be treatable. A disinhibited colon is frequently seen in dementia, especially later on, and can be controlled with a bowel regime if need be, but this is unpleasant. Containment in pads is often better, but poorly tolerated by carers. Incontinence is often the trigger for care home placement.

6. Pain is a symptom that requires diagnosis. The subtle and abstract thinking this requires on the part of the patient is often beyond someone with dementia, so the doctor needs to be alert and open-minded. Regular paracetamol is moderately effective and essentially side effect free, and forms the basis of all pain control regimens. If more is needed, tread the tightrope between desired and adverse effects, using weak or strong opiates, tramadol, or NSAIDs as appropriate.

7. Parkinsonism can be incidental to dementia, part of the syndrome of DLB, or arise through drug treatment or cerebrovascular disease. Dopamine agonists carry an unacceptable burden of neuropsychiatric side effects and are best avoided outside of very specialist hands. Avoid antimuscarinic drugs completely. Levodopa is better tolerated, but optimizing its use is difficult and may need the help of an interested neurologist, geriatrician, or nurse specialist. Motor symptoms in DLB respond to levodopa in 25% of cases.

8. Clinical decision-making demands open communication with patient and carers and a willingness of professionals to offer opinions that are realistic and humane rather than obsessive or defensive, whilst avoiding presumption and discrimination. Accept that sometimes you will make mistakes or miss things.

Palliative care in dementia

Definition of palliative care

'Palliative care is an approach that improves quality of life of patients and their families facing the problems associated with life threatening illness, through the prevention and relief of suffering by means of early identification and impeccable assessment and treatment of pain and other problems, physical, psychosocial and spiritual.' (WHO 2002)

'Palliating' is 'alleviation without curing'. It is not non-treatment or withdrawal of active treatments. Instead, it is a prioritization of treatments with the aim of relieving distress, minimizing burden related to treatment, and restoring what independence, autonomy, and control is possible in the circumstances.

You can quite legitimately argue that all management in dementia is 'palliative' by this definition. Here we discuss management anticipating death; although the process of dying may be very prolonged in dementia.

The extent of the problem

Surveys undertaken in many parts of the world suggest that care in the last phase of life can be improved.

Dementia is not a condition that can be cured; sometimes it is the main cause of death. Many of the general principles of good palliative care, developed for the management of people dying from cancer, are applicable in dementia. However, they are very different conditions. Mercifully, severe pain is rarely a major problem in advanced dementia; although people with dementia are less likely to be offered analgesia for predictably painful conditions than people without dementia.

People with dementia who are dying are nobody's specific responsibility. In the UK, most people with advanced dementia are resident in care homes, but staff there are often poorly trained for this work. Medical care falls to GPs, who may or may not have expertise in this time-consuming task. Secondary care psychiatric services may see their role as primarily to support people in the community rather than to be involved with terminal care. Patients may be admitted as medical emergencies to busy and disrupted admissions units more geared towards interventions to prolong life.

It is helpful to plan in advance what care people with dementia and their relatives will wish to receive in the final stages of the illness (📖 Chapter 11), but there will be many occasions when health and social care teams only become involved in a crisis.

The approach of death

By and large, people with dementia die of complications and comorbidities rather than the dementing illness itself.

As the disease progresses, patients become frailer—that is, they are both more functionally impaired and more vulnerable to deterioration. In particular:

• Immobility and its complications: orthostatic pneumonia, DVT and PE, and pressure sores.
• Falls and trauma, including hip fractures.
• Swallowing difficulties and appetite loss, leading to compromised nutrition and aspiration pneumonia.
• Proneness to infection due to age, poor nutrition, and communal living (e.g. influenza, other pneumonias, and diarrhoeal diseases).

In addition, people with dementia can suffer any of the other fatal illnesses that afflict older people—ischaemic heart disease (heart attack, heart failure), cancer, stroke, and chronic lung or kidney disease. Secondary prevention of vascular disease and help to stop smoking may not be seen as priorities for people with dementia. Many patients will still be offered annual influenza vaccination, in part to maintain 'herd immunity'.

Complications and comorbidities can strike at any time, but become more likely the frailer the patient becomes. Many intercurrent illnesses, especially infections, are successfully treated to the benefit of the patient. But by the time a patient has become severely affected, perhaps immobile, mute, and not recognizing family members, likelihood of response to treatment decreases, and the desirability of attempting curative therapy is open to question.

Without wanting to prejudge the issue one way or the other, even before the terminal phase, aggressive intervention (e.g. mechanical ventilation, chemotherapy, major surgery) for severe illnesses may or may not be desirable. The key is to address each individual's situation with an open mind and to come to a considered decision using the principles of benefit, burden, autonomy/best interests, and justice (📖 Chapter 12). In this context, justice includes not discriminating against someone just because they carry a label of 'dementia'. Having set out what is technically possible and the chances of success or otherwise, a useful question in discussions with families is 'What would he or she have wanted if they were able to tell us?' The answer will often be against 'aggressive' attempts at prolonging life.

Good medical care may involve recognizing that someone is approaching the end of their life and that palliative rather than potentially curative treatment is best. Doctors should ask themselves 'What are we aiming to achieve?' If the answer is most likely a prolongation of the process of dying, or survival in a distressed and distressing state, it is hard to argue that the proposed management will be successful. There are many value and judgement calls here, so open communication is vital. It is easier if this has been discussed in advance, at a stage of the illness where the patient can take some part.

Principles of palliative care

The key principles of palliative medicine are:
- Meticulous management of symptoms.
- Open communication.
- Psychological, emotional, and spiritual support of the patient and of those close to them.

Approach

Death in dementia usually comes after a prolonged period of ill health, and so has to be managed in the context of what has gone before:
- Inexorable loss of abilities.
- Good and bad experiences.
- Multiple hospital admissions.
- Carer strain.
- 'Anticipatory grief' (carers may already have grieved for the loss of the person they knew before dementia).
- Successful and unsuccessful changes of location.

An important part of the history is to clarify this.

Problems are likely to be a complex mix of physical, cognitive, behavioural, social, and professional. A problem list can help you manage the complexity (🕮 chapter 8 p. 199).

Management also follows the basic pattern set out in Chapter 8, under Treatment:
- Identify each symptom, issue, or disability—including practical arrangements for personal and nursing care and carer support.
- Explain, or diagnose, each problem:
- Intervene
  - set goals
  - cure pathologies
  - palliate symptoms
  - remediate disabilities
- Review the effect of the treatment.
- Anticipate: drug side effects or withdrawal, pressure sores and how to avoid them, family and carers' distress, what to do next time?
- Identify outstanding problems and make plans to manage them.
- Consider the best location for care:
  - is discharge home possible?
  - is a care home happy to oversee terminal care?

Problems with nutrition

Weight loss is common through the course of dementia, due to loss of appetite, the effects of drugs, or over-activity. Often by the time a person with dementia reaches the terminal phase they appear poorly nourished.

The first step, if possible, is to work out why. It could be a problem with:

- Appetite (and if so, why?).
- Cognition (forgetting to eat, or whether you have eaten).
- Swallowing (neurogenic or mechanical, dementia-related, or due to another condition such as stroke or Parkinson's disease).
- Comorbidity (cancer, infections including TB, any severe gastro-intestinal, heart, or lung disease).

Appetite failure

Appetite failure is common in advanced dementia and may be precipitated or exacerbated by acute illness. Look for drug causes of suppressed appetite (e.g. opiates) or nausea (many). Poor appetite may reflect constipation, depression, pain, hypothyroidism, hypercalcaemia, sepsis, or cancer. The assistance of dieticians and speech therapists who are interested in dementia can be reassuring to the family and the dementia team.

Nausea can be caused by renal failure, hypercalcaemia, hyponatraemia, and raised intra-cranial pressure.

Look also for a dry or sore mouth or denture problems.

Besides seeking and respecting food preferences, short courses of prednisolone 10–30 mg od or unlicensed use of megestrol 80–160 mg bd for 2 weeks in the first instance improve appetite in the short term, and sometimes 'kick start' it in the longer term.

Making swallowing safer

In the absence of a convincing 'medical' cause, feeding problems are initially managed by patient and skilled nursing to make swallowing as easy and safe as possible:

- Upright positioning.
- Changing the diet or its consistency (soft or blended, thickened fluids).
- Slow pacing—allowing each mouthful to be cleared before offering the next.
- Increasing frequency of meals.
- Giving liquid high-protein, high-energy food supplements.

Artificial nutrition and hydration (ANH)

As problems worsen, weight loss may become severe. The swallow reflex may become unsafe, allowing food and fluid to enter the trachea, causing choking, or recurrent infection (aspiration pneumonia). Swallowing may also become unsafe during an acute intercurrent illness or as a result of a stroke, with some potential for recovery.

Encouraging a good oral intake of food and fluids using diet supplements and pureed food is part of basic care, which is a fundamental human right and cannot be subject to a legal advance refusal. It is unlawful to deny the offer of food and drink, even if there is a danger of aspiration. However, using enteral and parenteral tubes to deliver nutrition and hydration is medical treatment ('artificial nutrition and hydration'), which like any other treatment can only be given with the patient's consent or under some other appropriate legal safeguard (📖 Chapter 11).

Clearly if any attempt at swallowing leads to distressing aspiration, it cannot be considered in anyone's interest. Most patients simply do not want to try to eat. Sips of water are unlikely to cause undue problems. Mouth care is especially important for any patient who is not swallowing.

Tube feeding may be via a nasogastric tube in the short term, or a percutaneous endoscopic gastrostomy (PEG) tube, which can potentially be maintained indefinitely. Nasogastric tubes are moderately uncomfortable to put in, may irritate whilst in, and are often pulled out. Once in, PEG tubes are more comfortable, easier to manage, and are generally problem free. Occasionally they are pulled out, the insertion site may become infected, they may block, or, if not periodically loosened and moved, they may become embedded in the gastric mucosa.

ANH is a form of life sustaining treatment and can be the subject of an advance decision, or decided by an attorney, if it has been specifically considered and documented in writing. However, less formal opinions can be taken into account as part of a best interest determination.

Evidence from the United States, where historically tube feeding has been used more aggressively than in the UK, suggests that the benefits of tube feeding are not great. Swallowing failure is usually a pre-terminal event. People with advanced dementia generally do not understand why they should be subject to these devices. A balance sheet of potential benefits and potential harm from ANH is given in Table 10.1. In general, we would not advocate tube feeding in advanced dementia. However, in each case the pros and cons will be differently balanced. Some people will have strongly held individual opinions.

The main problem in deciding on the desirability of tube feeding is *uncertainty*, about:

- Outcomes. By and large, dementia-related loss of swallowing is pre-terminal, and artificial hydration or nutrition is ineffective in prolonging life or delivering other benefits. However, swallowing may (or may not) recover after treatment of an intercurrent illness, or with time after a new stroke in vascular dementia.
- How people feel about the value or worth of the likely outcomes. Most (but not all) people consider life with severe dementia to be at least as bad as death.
- The quality of the evidence on which we have to base decisions. If someone has written an advance decision (living will) that anticipates the situation, there is little difficulty. Most have not. We are usually dependent on the opinions of family or friends, or a holder of a Power of Attorney, as to what the person would have wished.

Table 10.1 Benefits and drawbacks of ANH in terminal dementia

Potential good	Potential harm
Relieve thirst and hunger	Risk of death or complications during insertion of PEG
Prolong life	Prolong the process of dying
Ensure best chance of making a recovery	Survival in a distressing, highly dependent state
Minimize muscle catabolism, preserving muscle mass	Loss of dignity
Ease of nursing	

The same arguments about the desirability of feeding tubes apply to intravenous and subcutaneous fluids (except that these options have to be regularly reconsidered, as cannulae must be re-sited from time to time).

BMA guidelines suggest that decisions to withhold or withdraw feeding or hydration should be subject to a second consultant opinion. This would be desirable in an ideal world, especially where patients have not made advanced care plans.

Health care workers are sometimes reluctant to embark on procedures such as artificial nutrition and hydration because of a fear that once treatment has been started they will be liable to legal action if it is then stopped. The general advice from legal and ethical experts is that it is quite appropriate to withdraw treatment of this kind if it is shown that it is not benefiting the patient.

Immobility

Immobility

- Most people with severe dementia 'go off their feet'.
- This may make care easier if the risk of wandering or falling is reduced.
- There is often a difficult phase when the person is able to get out of the chair, but is not able to maintain standing balance.
- Appropriately designed seating may be helpful here, providing a 'gentle' form of restraint (perhaps more 'discouragement' than restraint), but close observation is essential.
- There may be times when it is appropriate to consider more overt physical restraint. This should only be considered:
  - where the person is at serious risk of falls
  - when they cannot be involved in activity to distract them from risky behaviour
  - where family, friends, or (for the unbefriended) an advocate agree that this is the best course of action
  - where the person with dementia acquiesces in the restraint adopted and does not attempt to resist or escape.
  - The RCN guideline Restraint Revisited (www.rcn.org) offers helpful guidance.
- Passive extension of limbs may help to prevent the development of flexion contractures.
- People who are immobile are at increased risk of infections, particularly of the soft tissues, chest, and urinary tract.
- Poor posture can also cause swallowing difficulties and the risk of aspiration.
- Occupational therapists, physiotherapists, and speech and language therapists can help with this (📖 Chapter 5).

Risk of injury to carers

Immobility also places a huge physical burden on carers and there is a real risk of physical injury. Paid carers are covered by health and safety legislation that applies across Europe. This law compels employers to educate workers in safe manual handling techniques and to provide any necessary lifting equipment. In essence this means 'no lifting'. Unfortunately the necessary equipment is generally not well-designed for people who cannot co-operate with being hoisted.

Informal carers are not bound by manual handling regulations and they often put their own health at risk in the effort to provide care as the person with dementia wishes. Carer education should include guidance on safe manual handling techniques.

Neurological problems

- Seizures can occur in later stages of dementia. When they occur out of the blue they can be terrifying for carers. Myoclonus (sudden muscular jerking) may be a pointer that major seizures are imminent.
- Fits do not always require treatment. Sometimes the adverse effects of antiepileptic medication are worse than the seizures.
- If fits are occurring frequently or causing great distress, sodium valproate is generally well tolerated. Start at 200 mg bd or tds (or MR 500 mg od) and increase slowly (over weeks) until control is achieved. Valproate can cause nausea, weight gain, and hair loss.
- Myoclonus is particularly common in DLB. Clonazepam is generally effective and free from serious adverse effects, but it often causes sedation. Start at 500 mcg *nocte*, increase slowly up to a maximum of 4 mg/day. Sodium valproate or lamotrigine are alternatives.

Infection

If someone is inevitably about to die, antibiotics serve no purpose, unless they are intended to relieve distressing symptoms. They will not usually form part of good terminal care.

The principles of benefit, burden, and autonomy should underlie decisions to commence antibiotic treatment (the framework should be held in mind even if the process is not explicitly followed).

Antibiotic treatment for pneumonia is best thought of in terms of probabilities rather than the more usual black and white. It is not a matter of 'active treatment—survival' versus 'no active treatment—death'. Rather, it is '20% chance of survival without treatment' versus '60% chance of survival with treatment'. Oxygen or opiates may relieve the distress of dyspnoea (but many people with dementia do not tolerate an oxygen mask or nasal cannulae).

Urinary tract infections are common, and are difficult to eradicate if fluid intake is poor or if there is a urinary catheter.

One consequence of opting not to treat intercurrent infections on the grounds that the patient is terminally ill is that the patient survives, but is further debilitated. Decisions about use of antibiotics are often determined by the degree of distress that the infection is causing.

Antibiotics have a downside, especially where *Clostridium difficile* is endemic. *C. difficile* colitis is a debilitating, long lasting, and difficult to treat diarrhoea that severely undermines quality of life.

Pain management

- Pain management is described in Chapter 9.
- In terminal care, get control of the pain quickly. The drug you choose depends on initial severity. Use oral morphine or subcutaneous diamorphine if necessary, and then decide on a regular regime.
- Give analgesics regularly for constant or recurring pain. Prescribe short-acting medication as required for acute exacerbations in spite of regular analgesia ('breakthrough pain').

The ladder of pain relief

- Always give paracetamol 1 g qds.
- Consider non-pharmacological treatment: heat/ice; massage; acupuncture; TENS.
- Non-steroidal anti-inflammatory drugs: ibuprofen 400 mg tds; diclofenac 50 mg tds.
- 'Weak opiates' (dihydrocodeine, codeine, tramadol). None is well tolerated by confused older people and they should generally be avoided.
- Low-dose strong opiates: dose morphine (e.g. MR 10 mg bd) or transdermal buprenorphine (5–20 mcg/h).
- Strong opiates e.g. morphine MR 20 mg bd po, or 5–10 mg 4 hourly SC or IM, diamorphine 2.5–5 mg 4 hourly SC or IM:
  - All patients on strong opiates become constipated. Stimulant laxatives may need to be given several times a day. Use senna, 2 tablets (15 mg) od or bd, or co-danthramer, initially 2 capsules at night, plus docusate sodium 200 mg bd as a stool softener. Add a macrogol (e.g. Movicol®) if necessary.
  - 30–50% of patients on strong opiates get nausea, but it is transient (give cyclizine 50 mg tds, metoclopramide 10 mg tds, or haloperidol 1–2 mg/day for first week).
  - Drowsiness is also usually transient (few days).
  - Dry mouth is common.
  - Other opiate-induced problems include: hallucinations (try a different opiate or give haloperidol); vivid dreams; myoclonus (use clonazepam); gastric stasis; itch.
- Alternative opiates:
  - buprenorphine patches (applied for 7 days at a time, steady state in 24 h, low or high dose, 5–35 mcg/h making for easy titration)
  - fentanyl patches (applied for 3 days at a time, steady state in 12–24 h, less constipating than morphine. Start with the smallest patch 12 mcg/h)
  - oxycodone (MR start at 10 mg bd; less drowsiness and delirium than morphine, fewer dreams and hallucinations, available rectally).

Tolerance is a minor problem. Addiction is defined as an overpowering drive to take a drug for its psychological effects, associated with behaviours such as drug seeking, escalating doses, loss of social control, and neglect of personal hygiene. Addiction does not occur with drugs taken for pain control; patients and relatives can be reassured of this.

- Pains that respond poorly or only partly to opiates include:
  - neuropathic pain (try pregabalin or amitriptyline)
  - bone pain (add a non-steroidal anti-inflammatory drug, radio-therapy)
  - raised intra-cranial pressure (use dexamethasone)
  - tension headache (paracetamol, non-steroidal anti-inflammatory drugs)
  - muscle cramp.

Routes of drug administration

The oral route is often not available because people dying with dementia are either drowsy or unable to swallow.

- Rectal absorption is good. Paracetamol, diclofenac, domperidone, and carbamazepine are available.
- Transdermal fentanyl, buprenorphine, and hyoscine hydrobromide (1 mg/72 hours) are available.
- Transmucosal lorazepam and prochlorperazine are available.
- Subcutaneous (use a 22G butterfly needle). Metoclopramide, cyclizine, hyoscine butylbromide, haloperidol, and diamorphine can all be used.
- Syringe drivers are useful, especially in the agonal (immediately pre-death) phase.

Cardiopulmonary resuscitation

When cardiac arrest occurs in people with terminal dementia it is rare for the cause to be ventricular fibrillation or tachycardia. Sudden cardiac death in dementia is most likely to be due to pulseless electrical activity or pulmonary embolism. It follows that even impeccably performed cardio-pulmonary resuscitation is unlikely to succeed.

There may be a case for teaching CPR to staff caring for people with dementia, but these skills are most likely to be useful away from the workplace. Still, some families are extraordinarily reluctant to accept that attempting CPR is a futile and undignified procedure.

Transfer to acute hospital

Care homes and other long stay institutions must include in a resident's care plan when transfer from the home to an acute unit may be beneficial. Advanced decisions about this must be observed.

Care home residents should not automatically be denied the benefits of modern medicine; for example it will rarely be possible for fractures to be adequately treated without orthopaedic surgery.

Treatment of acute infections and other medical conditions will often be possible in a care home. Transfer to hospital is distressing not only to people with dementia and their families, but also to other patients at the acute hospital.

The criterion should be that transfer should be arranged when what is needed and wanted cannot be otherwise provided.

Terminal care

'Terminal care' is the management of patients in whom the advent of death is felt to be certain and not far off. For these patients, medical effort is wholly directed at relief of symptoms and psychological support of patient and family, rather than cure or prolongation of life.

Does symptom control hasten death?

- Palliative care intends neither to hasten nor postpone death.
- Good symptom control may extend rather than shorten life.
- If symptom control measures do shorten life, this is permissible in UK law if the intention is relief of suffering rather than expediting death (the principle of double effect, *R v Bodkin Adams* [1956] Crim LR 265—an act which is foreseen to have both good and bad effects is legitimate, provided the act itself is good or at least neutral, the good effect is not caused by the bad effect, and the bad is proportionate to the good).
- Motivation and proportionality are hard to judge. If the sole reason for doing something is to hasten death, it is both illegal and wrong.

The last few days of life

- Encourage participation by the patient's family and friends in decision-making and practical care, according to their views and wishes.
- Reassess needs. Look for non-verbal signs of distress (agitation, grimacing, groaning), examine possible sites of pain (mouth, heels).
- Treat distressing symptoms and stop all other medication. Pain can always be controlled, but sometimes at the cost of drowsiness or continual sleep.
- Use morphine or diamorphine subcutaneously, intermittently, or by syringe driver. If the patient has not had opiates before, start at 5–10 mg/24 h. If opiates have been used before, the dose will depend on previous doses, response, body build, and renal function. Transdermal opiates (fentanyl, buprenorphine) are alternatives but take a day or two to act maximally.
- Other drugs can be added to a syringe driver according to the clinical situation, and may include:
  - haloperidol (initially 2.5 mg/24 h) for nausea or agitation
  - midazolam (initially 10 mg/24 h) for anxiety or fitting
  - hyoscine butylbromide (60 mg/24 h) for retained respiratory secretions
  - Levomepromazine (start at 5–25 mg/24 h) is a powerful antiemetic and sedative, which may also be analgesic and can be given subcutaneously. Sedation is usual with doses above 50 mg/day
  - Some of these are non-licensed indications.
- Prescribe as required medication for anticipated symptoms—agitation, anxiety, pain, convulsions, noisy respiratory secretions.
- Stop routine observations and investigations unless there is a specific problem to solve, which enhances comfort.

- Dry mouth is caused by mouth breathing, drugs, and/or poor fluid intake. Parenteral fluids are rarely needed. Dehydration is not painful and patients rarely complain of thirst. Continued hydration may increase the distress of dying. Use local measures to relieve dry mouth. These must be done regularly and assiduously. Relatives can usefully help in doing this.
- Allow access to water or food by mouth if this is wanted.
- Continue skin care and containment of incontinence—use a sheath or pads or a catheter if necessary.
- Assess relatives' needs.

If the patient is unconscious, or nearly so, and shows no signs of distress, some treatments that are neutral in terms of benefit or harm to the patient can be justified if they help relieve distress in relatives. Examples include a 'cosmetic' subcutaneous fluid infusion, hyoscine for excessive respiratory secretions, and diamorphine or haloperidol for agitation or restlessness.

Going home to die

In the last phase of dementia, care issues are sometimes very different from those in the middle stages of the condition. Over-activity and aggression are often replaced by apathy, immobility, and sleepiness.

An environment that was appropriate for a boisterous and mobile person may be less suitable for one who is becoming increasingly dependent. Although it is not always a good idea to move people with advanced dementia, this can sometimes be beneficial. Some families may wish to take their relatives home. They often cope better with physical care than challenging behaviour, and with specialized intensive home terminal care to support this.

A care home that sees management of psychological difficulties as its main role may not be adequately provided with specialized equipment for a person who is immobile with fragile skin. Sadly, funding bodies may insist on moving a person who has been housed in a specialized unit if the condition that required specialized care is no longer present.

Psychological and spiritual support—patients and families

Psychological assessment and management for people dying with dementia is all the more difficult because of confusion, drowsiness, and dysphasia. In many cases there will be no meaningful verbal communication between the patient and staff or family.

Communication is the cornerstone of effective psychological support. This comprises listening and talking. Good communication saves time and is more satisfying and less stressful. Tailor the giving of information to the wishes and understanding of the recipient, especially that involving bad news.

Be empathic. Empathy is putting yourself in someone else's shoes. If we have not been in a similar situation ourselves, we must use our imaginations. But people differ one from another, so not everyone's feelings and emotions will be the same as yours. Recognize both the distress of dying or seeing a close relative die, and of being in a strange and disempowering environment (a hospital or care home).

A drowsy person who is not agitated probably has no distress, but it is difficult to be sure. Hearing is said to be the last of the senses to be lost. Assume that drowsy patients can hear, and welcome attention and company. Don't talk as if they are not there. Reassure relatives that their presence is helpful, even when they seem to be getting little response in return. Encourage staff not to neglect patients because routine observations have been stopped.

Spirituality may become especially important in the last phase; it may help to put the experience of dying and dementia in a broader perspective.

Most people fear death, but many older people are remarkably philosophical about it. They realize that lifespan is not infinite, and will have seen contemporaries die. If the patient is able to engage, you can assume that they will have thought about their own death in general terms. Many dying patients are aware of what is happening and can understand and accept.

Summary

1. People with dementia deserve appropriate care when they are dying.
2. Swallowing failure, like other symptoms, should be assessed and diagnosed. In advanced dementia it is usually a pre-terminal event, and artificial hydration and nutrition are unlikely to be of benefit.
3. It is often difficult to be sure when people with advanced dementia are experiencing distress and what the cause of their distress is. In particular, pain is often missed or under-treated.
4. Many conventional medical treatments may be inappropriate for people with advanced dementia.
5. If death is thought to be not far off, reassess needs. Prioritize measures to control symptoms and maintain dignity, rather than those aimed at prevention or prolongation of life. Consider if a discharge home is desirable or possible.

Chapter 11

Legal aspects of dementia care

Legal aspects of capacity

Caring for a person with dementia may involve performing many acts that in other circumstances could be regarded as illegal. Even touching someone without their consent might constitute an assault, so there are potential difficulties in bathing, dressing, or administering medication to a person who lacks capacity to consent to these procedures. In almost all countries there are laws to authorize such care. This chapter is written in the light of UK legislation, specifically that for England and Wales. Northern Ireland has no incapacity law at present, but the government has announced its intention to introduce a measure based on the English Mental Capacity Act (MCA). The wording in the Scottish Adults with Incapacity Act (AWI) is somewhat different but the underlying principles are virtually identical.

The definition of capacity to make a decision is given in Box 11.1.

The law lays down basic principles to be considered when deciding whether or not someone lacks capacity to make a decision (💷 Box 11.2); capacity relates to a specific decision and not to decisions in general.

Capacity is defined in law

- Capacity is defined in UK law by:
  - England and Wales Mental Capacity Act 2005
  - Scotland Adults with Incapacity Act 2000.
- Each is accompanied by a Code of Practice that cannot be ignored by professionals.
- Capacity relates to a specific decision at a specific time—it is not an all or nothing state.
- To come within this legal framework, lack of capacity must be due to:
  - impairment of, or disturbance in the functioning of, the mind or brain (England and Wales)
  - mental disorder or inability to communicate because of physical disorder (Scotland).
- Incapacity may result from a lack of education or information, but this is not covered by law.
- If there is dispute about whether a person has capacity to make a decision, this can be resolved by a court:
  - Court of Protection in England and Wales
  - Sheriff Court in Scotland.
- The Public Guardian oversees the administration of the law for people without capacity.

Box 11.1 Definition of capacity (from England and Wales MCA 2005)

A person is unable to make a decision for himself if he is unable:
(a) to understand the information relevant to the decision
(b) to retain that information
(c) to use or weigh that information as part of the process of making the decision, or
(d) to communicate his decision (whether by talking, using sign language, or any other means).

The fact that a person is able to retain the information relevant to a decision for a short period only does not prevent him from being regarded as able to make the decision.

The information relevant to a decision includes information about the reasonably foreseeable consequences of:
(a) deciding one way or the other, or
(b) failing to make the decision.

Box 11.2 Principles (from England and Wales MCA 2005)

- People are assumed to have capacity unless it is proved that they have not.
- A person is not to be regarded as unable to make a decision unless all practicable attempts to help him to do so have been taken without success.
- A person is not to be regarded as unable to make a decision because he makes an unwise decision.
- Any act done for a person who lacks capacity must be done in his best interests.
- The outcome cannot be achieved by less restrictive means.

If a person lacks capacity in respect of decision, then whoever makes a decision on their behalf must do so 'to their benefit' (Scotland) or 'in their best interests' (elsewhere in the UK). The essence of 'best interests' is summed up in Box 11.3. For people with dementia the key test is the third bullet point. The correct decision will be the one that the person would have wanted for themselves, if they were able to decide. Where the person previously had a learning disability and did not hold a strong opinion, other factors will need to be considered.

Personal and medical care

Personal care in England and Wales can legally be given under s.5 of the MCA (*Acts in relation to care and treatment*), which allows personal and medical care to be given in an appropriate manner without any need for legal formalities to be completed. This could include carers using money belonging to the person without capacity to buy necessary goods and services (📖 p. 294). Staff employed to give care may only act in the best interests of the person without capacity and must 'have regard to' the MCA Code of Practice when acting without explicit consent. It is also possible to use this procedure for necessary expenditure on behalf of a person lacking capacity (s.7 and s.8).

In Scotland (AWI s.47) a certificate has to be completed by the medical practitioner primarily responsible for the medical treatment of the adult.

Consent to medical treatment

Many people with dementia may retain the capacity to consent to aspects of their medical treatment (📖 Box 11.1). If a person has capacity, then the wishes of proxy decision-makers and the person's own advanced decisions on treatment are irrelevant. The process of obtaining agreement for treatment for a person who lacks capacity is shown in Figure 11.1.

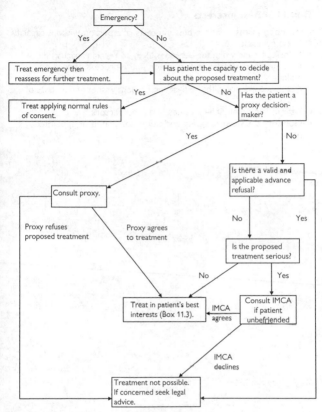

Fig. 11.1 Consent to treatment flowchart.

Notes to flowchart:

Proxy decision-makers include holders of Lasting Powers of Attorney for health and welfare and court appointed deputies (England and Wales), and holders of Continuing Power Attorney and Welfare Guardians in Scotland.

IMCA—Independent Mental Capacity Advocate (📖 p. 294).

The flowchart does not apply to treatment decisions made under mental health legislation.

Box 11.3 Best interests

In order to assess what the best interests of a person without capacity are, it is necessary to:
- Consider if and when the person is likely to regain capacity.
- Maximize participation of the person in the process of decision-making.
- Act in accordance with the past and present wishes and feelings of the person.
- Bear in mind their beliefs, values, and other factors.
- Consider the views of carers and other nominated or appointed persons.

Planning for future incapacity

Planning for future incapacity

Advance decisions to refuse treatment

- In England and Wales the MCA sections 24–26 specify how to make a legally binding advance decision refusing treatment.
- If the decision is about life-sustaining treatment, it must be made in writing in a prescribed format.
- There is no specified form for refusal of other treatments.
- It must be made by a person who is 18 or over and at a time when the person has capacity to make it.
- It must specify the treatment that is being refused, although this can be in lay terms (for example using 'tummy' instead of abdomen).
- It may specify particular circumstances, again in lay terms, in which the refusal will apply.
- A person can change or completely withdraw the advance decision, so long as they have capacity to do so—this does not need to be in writing.

Additional requirements for refusal of life-sustaining treatment

- An advance decision will not apply to life-sustaining treatment unless it is verified by a statement confirming that the decision is to apply even if life is at risk.
- Both the decision and the statement verifying it must be in writing, must be signed, and the signature must be witnessed. The person making the advance directive may instruct another person to sign it on their behalf in their presence.
- The person does not physically need to write the advance decision themselves.
- Advance decisions recorded in medical notes are considered to be in writing.
- Writing can also include electronic records.

Advance decision exceptions

An advance refusal is not valid if:
- The person has withdrawn the decision at a time when they had capacity.
- They subsequently make a welfare LPA, appointing someone else to make the relevant decision.
- They have done anything that is inconsistent with the advance refusal.

It is not applicable if:
- The treatment is not the treatment specified in the advance decision.
- Any circumstances specified in the advance decision are absent.
- There are reasonable grounds for believing that circumstances exist that the person did not anticipate at the time of the advance decision, which would have affected their decision had they anticipated them.

Guidance for health and social care professionals on advance refusals is contained in Chapter 9 of the Code of Practice. If there is doubt as to whether an advance directive exists, or whether it is valid or applicable, an approach should be made to the relevant court. Urgent treatment may be given whilst awaiting a decision from the court.

In Scotland, advance directives do not form part of the Adults with Incapacity Act. However, in s.275 and s.276 of the Scottish Mental Health (Care and Treatment) Act (MHCTSA), there are provisions to allow people who have capacity to make written, witnessed statements about the treatment they may wish to receive for future mental disorder at a time when they do not have the capacity to make their own decisions on treatment.

Wishes and feelings

The provisions of the MCA only apply to refusals of treatment. It is not possible to make binding advance requests for treatment; there is no requirement for a doctor to provide treatment for a patient that would not—in the doctor's opinion—be appropriate for the patient.

The specific provisions for the making of advance decisions are difficult to operationalize; it is not clear how widely they will be used. However, it is often helpful to get some idea of the treatments that people with dementia would wish to have after they have lost capacity to express their feelings. All too often, decision-making is compromised (or paralysed) by lack of this information. Insofar as advance decision documents give a general impression of values and opinions, or can be extrapolated to do so, they are useful. Usually we are reliant on views expressed to relatives or friends in undocumented conversations. Although it is usually easy enough to judge the veracity of these, the potential for abuse through misreporting of wishes and feelings does exist.

The MCA requires professionals proposing treatment for a person without capacity to take into account the wishes and feelings of that person when establishing their best interests. It is good practice to make a record of such wishes in care plans produced under the Care Programme Approach or the Single Assessment Procedure. (Remember that advance decisions recorded in medical notes are considered to be in writing.) Specific regulations on this are in force in the MHCTSA.

Power of Attorney

People who are worried that at some time they may lose capacity to make their own decisions are able to appoint someone else—an 'attorney'—to act on their behalf.

- Powers of Attorney under capacity legislation are created by people (donors) who have the capacity to do so.
- They are known as Lasting Powers of Attorney (LPAs) in England and Wales, and Continuing or Welfare Powers of Attorney (CPAs) in Scotland.
- There are two types of Power of Attorney:
  - LPA for property and affairs, (Scotland Continuing Power of Attorney) dealing with financial matters
  - LPA for personal welfare (Scotland-Welfare Power of Attorney), dealing with health and social care issues.
- Only individuals can deal with health and welfare matters but firms can act as property and affairs attorneys.

- Only property and affairs LPAs can be used for a person who has capacity to make their own decisions.
- LPAs must be registered with the Office of the Public Guardian before use.
- They must be accompanied by a certificate from a designated person to confirm that the donor has capacity to execute an LPA.
- Registered health and social care practitioners may act as certificate providers. They need to certify that:
  - the donor understands the nature of the LPA and the powers they are giving
  - the donor has not been put under pressure to make the LPA
  - they are not aware of any other reasons why the LPA should not be created.
- Before LPAs and CPAs can be registered, people nominated by the donor must be notified and have the opportunity to object.
- Attorneys must always act 'in the best interests of' or 'to the benefit of' the adult without capacity.

Before the MCA came into force it was possible to make an Enduring Power of Attorney (EPA). They work in much the same way as an LPA for property and affairs. Existing EPAs are still valid, but new ones cannot be created.

The Offices of the Public Guardian (OPG) (www.publicguardian.gov.uk/ for England; www.publicguardian-scotland.gov.uk for Scotland) provide guidance for attorneys.

Appointed decision-makers

Deputies and guardians

If no attorney has been appointed, the Court of Protection in England and Wales, or the Sheriff Court in Scotland, may appoint someone with a specified role in decision-making to act as a 'deputy' in England and Wales or a 'guardian' in Scotland. Going to court to seek the appointment of a deputy is expensive and deputies must pay fees for supervision. The Office of the Public Guardian maintains a register of attorneys and deputies. It is possible for anyone to approach the OPG to establish whether a deputy or attorney has been appointed, but only those with a need to know may be told the details of any conditions that have been imposed on their decision-making.

Deputies and guardians may be appointed for either health and welfare decisions, or property and affairs, or both.

Appointees

It is possible to create an 'appointee' to collect the state benefits of people who cannot manage their own financial affairs. This includes old age pension, attendance allowance etc. An appointee may be either an individual person or the representative of an organization, such as a solicitor or a care home proprietor. This procedure is governed by the Social Security Claims and Payments Regulations 1987. If a person with dementia cannot manage their finances and has only limited funds, using this mechanism may avoid the expense of applying to the courts for a deputy or guardian. (See paragraphs 5000–5457 of the Department for Work and Pensions Online Guide, www.dwp.gov.uk/advisers/docs/aaarg/).

Other financial arrangements

The informal mechanisms of MCA s.5 (Acts in connection with care or treatment) may be used to pay for necessary goods and services (📖 Code of Practice paragraph 6.56–6.66).

There is no similar provision in Scotland, although managers of care homes can apply to manage their residents' funds under the Adults with Incapacity (Management of Residents' Finances) (Scotland) Act 2000.

Independent Mental Capacity Advocates

If a person without capacity has no relatives or friends who are taking an interest in their well-being, it may be necessary to seek the views of an Independent Mental Capacity Advocate. This is necessary:
- If an NHS body or Local Authority is proposing to place them in a care home or long-term hospital placement.
- If an NHS body is proposing 'serious medical treatment'. This is defined as:
  (a) in a case where a single treatment is being proposed, there is a fine balance between its benefits to the patient and the burdens and risks it is likely to entail for them

(b) in a case where there is a choice of treatments, a decision as to which one to use is finely balanced, or
(c) what is proposed would be likely to involve serious consequences for the patient.
- IMCAs may also be needed where there is concern that the person's relatives or friends may be subjecting them to abuse and where Vulnerable Adults procedures (☐ Chapter 5 p. 130) are being instituted.

Specific tests of capacity

There are a number of specific tests of capacity that have legal force:
- Make a will.
- Make a gift.
- Enter litigation.
- Enter into a contract.
- Deal with finances.
- Vote.
- Enter personal relationships.
- Consent to research and innovative treatment.

Most of these are beyond the scope of this book but it is helpful to know of the tests for capacity to make a will (testamentary capacity) (Box 11.4).

A person making a will must:
- Understand the nature and purpose of a will.
- Be aware of what their assets are and their approximate value.
- Be aware of people to whom they might be expected to make bequests.
- Be free from delusions that might cloud their judgement.
- Be able to express their wishes.

It is possible for the Court of Protection to make a Statutory Will on behalf of a person who lacks testamentary capacity. This can be done in retrospect after their death.

For further details of tests for capacity and their application see: *Assessment of Mental Capacity: Guidance for Doctors and Lawyers*, 2nd edition 2004. London: BMJ Publishing Group.

Box 11.4 Testamentary capacity

Banks v Goodfellow [1870] 5LR QB 549:

- 'A testator shall understand the nature of the act and its effects;
- shall understand the nature of the property of which he is disposing;
- shall be able to comprehend and appreciate the claims to which he ought to give effect;
- no disorder of mind shall poison his affections, pervert his sense of right, or prevent the exercise of his natural faculties;
- no insane delusion shall influence his will in disposing of his property.'

Deprivation of liberty

The European Convention on Human Rights (ECHR) specifies that no person shall be deprived of their liberty. There are exceptions to this, such as lawful imprisonment. Another exception is for 'people of unsound mind, in accordance with a procedure prescribed by law'. There must be legal procedures to authorize this.

Sometimes admitting a person with dementia to a hospital or care home will constitute deprivation of their liberty. The European Court of Human Rights recognizes that it may sometimes be necessary to restrict someone's liberty without prior legal formalities, but 'deprivation' of liberty needs formal authorization. There remains much uncertainty in legal circles about exactly where 'restriction of liberty' becomes 'deprivation of liberty'.

Compulsory admission to hospital under Mental Health Legislation

We always hope that people will accept our professional guidance on their treatment. However, there are some times when people with dementia need to be taken to hospital against their wishes, either to provide them with care that cannot otherwise be arranged or to protect other people from harm.

Dementia and delirium are mental disorders, so mental health legislation can be used in the situation where admission is necessary:

• in the interests of the patient's own health, or
• in the interests of the patient's own safety, or
• with a view to the protection of other persons.

Different sections of the England and Wales Mental Health Act (MHA) and Scottish MHCTSA authorize compulsory admission for varying periods (📖 Table 11.1). For most compulsory admissions ('sections'), two doctors, one with a previous knowledge of the patient and one with recognized expertise in psychiatry, must confirm that the conditions for detention are met. A specially trained social or health care practitioner ('approved mental health professional', AMHP) usually makes the application. The MHA specifies the professional training and required competencies required to be granted AMHP status. At present most AMHPs are social workers who have undergone special training in mental health. Approved doctors are mostly senior psychiatrists (although it is possible for GPs and others to be approved); they are required to undergo further training in mental incapacity if they are to undertake deprivation of liberty assessments.

Patients detained under the MHA may be treated with medication against their wishes. These powers may override those in capacity law. (📖 Mental Health Act Code of Practice). A relative or other named person can ask for the detained person to be discharged, and the person themselves has the right to apply to a tribunal to rule on whether detention is needed. Under certain circumstances, compulsory treatment in the community can be provided under mental health law. For further details, refer to the relevant Act and Code of Practice.

Table 11.1 Detention under British mental health legislation

	England and Wales (MHA)	Scotland (MHCTSA)
Emergency (72 hours)	s.4, s.5(2)	s.36
Assessment (28 days)	s.2	s.44
Treatment (6 months)	s.3	s.63

Mental health legislation can authorize supervised medical treatment in the community, and in England and Wales guardians may be appointed who have the power to specify where the subject of a guardianship order may live. Guardians can also require them to attend for medical treatment.

Deprivation of Liberty Safeguards (DoLS)

In 2005 the European Court of Human Rights declared that the UK was in breach of the ECHR by preventing the carers of a person without capacity from removing him from hospital even though he appeared content to stay. As an informal patient he did not have access to a tribunal. This judgement in the *Bournewood* case came after a long series of hearings through the UK courts and has had profound implications for many people with dementia in care homes and hospitals. A new procedure of authorization for deprivation of liberty has been set up to fill this gap in the law.

The onus to apply for authorization rests on the manager of the care home or the hospital in which the person is placed. They must apply to the 'Supervisory Body' for authorization. The Supervisory Body is the relevant local authority for care homes, and the commissioning authority, usually a Primary Care Trust, for hospitals. The regulations suggest that managers should seek authorization prior to the admission of a person without capacity, although it is difficult to see how a person with dementia might be able to judge in advance whether they would wish to agree to stay in a place that they have not experienced. In an emergency a 7 day order may be issued to allow time for a full assessment to take place.

There are two types of assessor who each need to undertake an approved course of training. Mental Health assessors are doctors, best interests assessors may be social workers nurses, OTs or psychologists.

Six separate assessments are required to authorize deprivation of liberty (📖 Box 11.5).

Box 11.5 England and Wales regulations on assessor's roles

Assessment	Carried out by
Age	Best interests assessor
Mental health	Mental health assessor
Mental capacity	Best interests or mental health assessor
Best interests	Best interests assessor
Eligibility	Best interests or mental health assessor
No refusals	Best interests assessor

A "refusal" would be;
– Opposition by a welfare deputy
– Opposition by the holder or a welfare LPA.
– The existence of a valid and applicable advance directive refusing treatment
The eligibility assessment is to ensure that the DoLS authorization does not conflict with any Mental Health Act requirement, and that use of the Mental Health Act would not be more appropriate. A DoLS authorization cannot be used to impose treatment for mental disorder on a hospital patient who is objecting to the treatment
   There is a supplement to the Mental Capacity Act Code of Practice covering the DoLS procedures.

There must be at least two assessors, the mental health and best interests assessors must be different people, and there must be no conflict of interest.

Concluding note
The law in this area is new and it is not clear how judges will interpret it in practice. It is always better to anticipate that people with dementia will progress to the point where they will not be able to make decisions for themselves and encourage them to make advance arrangements about what they would like to be done for them when they lose capacity to decide for themselves.

Sexual offences

The Sexual Offences Act 2003 was introduced to prevent the sexual exploitation of vulnerable people. According to s.27 of this Act:

(1) A person (A) commits an offence if:
   (a) he intentionally touches another person (B)
   (b) the touching is sexual
   (c) B is unable to refuse because of or for a reason related to a mental disorder, and
   (d) A knows or could reasonably be expected to know that B has a mental disorder and that because of it or for a reason related to it B is likely to be unable to refuse.

(2) B is unable to refuse if:
   (a) he lacks the capacity to choose whether to agree to the touching (whether because he lacks sufficient understanding of the nature or reasonably foreseeable consequences of what is being done, or for any other reason), or
   (b) he is unable to communicate such a choice to A.

The MCA does not include any measures that allow a proxy to consent to sexual relationships on behalf of a person who lacks capacity, so this means that it is illegal for a person who lacks capacity to consent to participate in any behaviour that is 'sexual'.

Sensitive discussions to establish what a person with impaired capacity might have wished in the relevant situation can be useful to guide management (📖 Chapter 4).

Summary

1. People with capacity may appoint others (attorneys) to make decisions for them if in the future they lose the ability to decide for themselves. They may also make advance refusals of treatment.

2. Courts can appoint decision-makers to act on behalf of people without capacity if they do not have attorneys.

3. It is lawful to provide basic care for somebody lacking capacity without any specific authorization.

4. Where people who lack capacity to consent are kept in care homes or hospitals their detention must be in their best interests and in accordance with the law.

5. There are specific legal safeguards for people without capacity.

Chapter 12

Making decisions

Decisions in dementia

Normally medical encounters run as follows: the patient notices a problem (or presents for prevention or screening), asks for medical help, therapeutic options are suggested (or reassurance given), and the patient decides whether to accept them or not.

In dementia (or delirium) things are different. The patient may or may not realize there is a problem, or accept it. They may or may not understand or be able to retain the diagnosis given, the therapeutic options offered, or the implications of accepting or declining. They may lack decision-making ability, which leads to questions about whether someone else should take decisions on behalf of the patient. If so, who (relative, other carer, or professional)?

Fortunately an ethical framework to guide us through these questions has evolved, and has been incorporated into law in the UK and elsewhere (☐ Chapter 11). The details vary between different jurisdictions, even within the UK, but the underlying principles are widely applicable.

Importantly, what is decided in any given situation can vary from one individual to another. There may be no clear 'right' answer, but it is important that the process of deciding is gone through correctly. UK law also allows for people to make legally binding decisions about how they wish to be cared for in the future and who they would like to make decisions on their behalf if the time comes when they cannot decide for themselves.

In this chapter we discuss practical aspects of decision-making.

Decisions for the future

The average survival after diagnosis for a person with dementia is 3–4 years for a man and 4–5 years for a woman—but this will clearly depend on age at diagnosis (☐ Chapter 18).

- Many sorts of agreement, including medical interventions, the making of contracts or wills, and everyday activities (shopping, paying bills, taking out insurance, having sexual relations) require decision-making capacity to be present, sometimes as part of a consent-giving process.
- At the time of diagnosis the person with dementia will often, but not always, have capacity to make decisions (or may be able to make some but not others).
- Soon after diagnosis it is necessary to think about how they want to be treated if (or when) they deteriorate and are no longer able to decide for themselves, or are unable to communicate.
- Making financial provisions (wills and property and affairs powers of attorney) are sensible precautions for anybody who may one day lose capacity—and that means all of us.
- Welfare powers of attorney (☐ Chapter 11) are useful in many situations, provided the person with dementia has a relative or friend who they trust, and who is prepared to take on the role of proxy decision-maker (realizing that this may become quite an onerous duty).
- Anticipating other losses may also be sensible. If moving into sheltered housing is considered, it is best to move as soon as possible so as to adapt to new surroundings whilst cognition is still reasonably good.
- Giving up driving early and using alternative transport may avoid greater tensions later on (☐ Chapter 5 p. 132).

- Advance decisions (living wills) have a place, but it can be hard to contemplate future situations in which they might apply. Advanced planning is much to be encouraged, but probably only individuals who feel strongly are likely to make legally binding arrangements.
- Remember that it may be distressing for both patients and relatives to go through possible scenarios of advanced dementia (📖 Chapters 7 and 10) when struggling to come to terms with a new diagnosis.

Capacity assessment in practice

The key issue in decision-making is that of mental capacity. The UK legal position on capacity is set out in Chapter 11.

Capacity is specific to a particular decision, and someone may be able to consent to some things but not others. In the UK, capacity is presumed to be present unless it is demonstrated to be lacking. With a diagnosis of dementia, capacity will always be in question and so must be assessed constantly, but without the process becoming unduly intrusive or disruptive.

Assessing capacity is asking whether someone can understand and weigh up information necessary to make a decision (🕮 Box 11.1). Specific 'tests' of capacity exist for various legal purposes, such as giving a power of attorney or making a will (🕮 Chapter 11).

Understanding need only be in broad terms. This is fortunate, as you might imagine that on these criteria a large proportion of patients cannot give their own consent.

Consent

Consent means agreement. Most health care interventions require consent. Merely touching someone without their permission may constitute 'battery'. Doing anything that might (to the legal mind) lead someone to fear an injury may be an assault. Health professionals are unused to thinking like this, but some patients, lawyers, and governments do.

The key points are:

- You must get consent before you examine, investigate, treat, or otherwise care for a competent adult patient.
- Consent may be *explicit* (permission asked and granted), or *implied* (the patient comes to you voluntarily, asks for help, co-operates, and does not object to what you are proposing or doing e.g. holding his or her arm out so you can take blood).
- Explicit consent can be written or verbal, and both are equally valid (although the latter is hard to prove without a witness).
- In the UK an adult is anyone over the age of 18 years.
- Capacity must be assessed separately for each decision. People may be competent to make some decisions but not others, and their ability to consent may vary with time. They may change their mind about consenting (or not consenting).
- A decision that you find surprising, or with which you disagree, does not prove that the person lacks capacity. Competent adults may refuse any treatment, even if it would clearly benefit their health, unless it is treatment of a mental illness and they are liable to detention under the Mental Health Act.
- Consent must be 'informed'—otherwise it is invalid. This means patients need sufficient information to be able to come to a decision, such as benefits and risks and possible alternative treatments. Reasonable support to help the person understand and decide must be given. This includes explanation in simple lay terms. Information leaflets produced by professional bodies should be used where they are available. Involve translators, deaf aids, and speech and language therapists as necessary.
- Consent must also be voluntary—not under any duress from relatives, friends, or staff.
- Consent may be obtained from another person who is legally authorized to do so. Alternatively, a person may be treated if it is in their 'best interests'. (📕 Box 11.3 and Fig. 11.1 p. 288).

How to make decisions

The dominant ethical framework currently is called 'Principalism'. This is widely applicable across different cultures and types of medical intervention. However, given its heavy emphasis on respect for autonomy, dementia is the condition where most problems arise.

Four elements are involved:
- Beneficence, or doing good ('benefits').
- Non-maleficence, or avoiding harm ('burdens or risks').
- Autonomy (or best interests).
- Justice, or equity.

The first two define whether an intervention is *effective* or not—is it technically feasible? Unless the likely good from a procedure outweighs the likely harm, or at least justifies it, it is not effective. Good and harm may be judged in terms of effect on length of life, curing diseases, reducing symptoms or increasing abilities, avoiding complications and side effects, and the short-term unpleasantness or debility associated with the procedure.

If a procedure is ineffective, or is highly unlikely to have its desired effect, it is said to be *futile*. In these cases consent is not generally an issue, as futile interventions should not be offered to patients. There may still be an obligation to give an explanation of why potential treatments are not being offered.

Assuming that there is a reasonable prospect of an intervention doing more good than harm, next consider autonomy. This is essentially the same as asking consent.

How you proceed depends on whether the patient has capacity to decide or not. A futile procedure should not be undertaken, even if a patient with capacity wants it, but otherwise the autonomy of competent patients must be respected. They can exercise it by refusing a treatment that might be effective. The only way of finding out what a patient wants is to ask them.

If a patient can give you the information you need, do not ask relatives or friends first. It is technically a breach of confidentiality to discuss things without the patient's permission, and opinions of relatives or friends may not accurately reflect those of the patient. If a patient does not have capacity, then we can still respect autonomy by trying to find out what they would have wanted.

Equity and justice refer to two things:
- *Non-discrimination*: on the basis of things that should have no influence on decision-making (sex, race, religion, political views, disability, age, cognitive function).
- *Rationing* (or fair shares): available resources must be used to maximize the good done overall to the greatest number of people. This is really the responsibility of politicians and health administrators. It can make life difficult for doctors, because the clinical ethic demands that we do our best for the patient in front of us, ideally without taking account of resource issues. As a general rule use common sense.

Best interests

The idea of 'best interests' applies where a patient does not have capacity to give or withhold consent, nor a legally valid substitute decision-maker. In the UK a treatment may be legally given, despite lack of consent, if it is in the patient's best interests (📖 Box 11.3). The issue of effectiveness still holds—the benefits of treatment must outweigh the burdens. There are several formulations of this from published documents that are useful when discussing the issues with involved parties (staff, relatives):

- Is the proposed treatment likely to lead to a length and quality of life that the patient would have found acceptable?
- Does the treatment make possible a decent life in which a patient can reasonably be thought to have a continued interest?

Both of these introduce ideas beyond the likely clinical outcome (length and quality of life). They include a need to respect the wishes of the patient. There are several levels of information:

- An advance decision, or living will, may legally define what the patient would or would not have wanted done. Advance decisions can only be used to refuse treatment. Unfortunately very few people have made these (have you?). Advance decisions are only legally binding if they are 'valid' and 'applicable'. There will often be some doubt as to whether the exact circumstances intended by the patient actually apply (📖 Chapter 11).
- A proxy judgement—the donee of a Welfare Lasting Power of Attorney, a court appointed welfare deputy, or an equivalent legally approved substitute decision-maker is a proxy. Even in the absence of a formally appointed decision-maker, someone may be able to tell you what the patient would have said, because they had discussed the issues previously. The degree of uncertainty mounts when the exact circum- stances have not been discussed, but opinions may still be known in general terms. This often comes down to asking 'knowing the person as you do, what do you think they would have wanted?'—which is a pretty rough and ready assessment of opinion.
- An expression of wishes may give an idea of what treatment the patient would like to receive. These may be recorded as part of the advanced care planning process. Unlike an advance refusal these are not binding but are helpful in determining whether a procedure may be in the patient's best interest.
- A substitute judgement—this asks what the informant (relative, friend, or staff member) would want in this situation. This may be useful when someone is of a particular religious faith, where general principles are well known. Staff making this judgement are essentially saying 'As a fellow human being what would I have wanted?' This has some validity, but opinions do vary widely.

Be careful, as research has shown that people with a condition tend to view it as less bad than do staff members, relatives, or members of the general population (who are the most averse to descriptions of severe disability). Some people rate living with dementia as bad as death, or worse than death. Many others disagree. Studies of quality of life have generally shown that people with dementia tend to rate their own quality of life quite highly.

Avoid giving the impression that you are asking family members to make life or death decisions. Unless they are legal proxies their decisions are not binding and it is unfair to burden families with further distress and possible guilt when they are having to cope with severe illness in a close relative. You are only asking what the patient would have wanted if they were able to give their opinion, and to satisfy your responsibilities under the Mental Capacity Act. The issue of 'emotional burden' on someone given a Lasting Power of Attorney and asked to make a life or death decision must be recognized, acknowledged, and supported (perhaps by offering to share the decision).

All this requires some knowledge about:
- The condition.
- Its natural history.
- The effectiveness of treatment.
- What the patient would have wanted you to do.

There is a degree of uncertainty about all of these, which can make life difficult and good judgement important. Fortunately the natural history of dementia is relatively predictable and there should be time for families to discuss in the early stages of the condition what will be best when the disorder becomes more severe and the person with dementia loses the capacity to make their own decisions.

Sometimes, uncertainty in decision-making means we must prevaricate. A holding operation for a few days (or weeks), such as intravenous hydration whilst we see which way things are turning out, is perfectly acceptable if a decision can be postponed. We are gathering more information on which to base a final judgement. This is in accordance with the principles of the Mental Capacity Act—that we should take the least restrictive action and before taking any action we must consider when capacity may be regained. Where the person has not appointed a proxy for health and welfare decisions when they had capacity to do so, it may be helpful to seek a court appointed deputy if a number of major decisions need to be made.

When the ethical framework is properly applied it is generally quite simple, and many nurses and junior doctors will have the necessary knowledge and skills. However, these discussions should usually involve the most senior doctor available. You should always be able to expect support, both in making decisions and discussing them or their consequences, if you need to.

Responsibility for deciding on best interest, and formally declaring it to be so, rests with the doctor in charge of the case. Senior staff may want support through discussing cases with colleagues or asking second opinions. For particularly difficult decisions, the advice of an ethics committee may be helpful.

Managing decision-making

The role of the professional

As health and social care professionals we must make decisions well, be seen to make them well, and 'carry' staff and families with us in the process. The ideal is to reach consensus and agreement. This is often possible by explaining the process behind decision-making and showing that we are not arbitrarily 'playing God'.

Sometimes, strong convictions and emotions raise barriers to what rational thought dictates. We must be sensitive to these—acknowledge them and show you understand them and take them into account.

• Remember, however, that acting against the 'best interests' of someone who cannot decide for themselves is an assault and is illegal.
• A 'cosmetic' course of antibiotics may help a relative come to terms with the impending death of a family member, and usually does little harm.
• Avoid being dogmatic, but you must always be ready and able to justify what you have done after the event.
• Common sense must prevail.

Advocates

Where there are disagreements between professionals and family and friends—or sometimes where there are fundamental differences between members of the care team—it is worth considering whether to seek an advocate to speak on behalf of the person with dementia or their carers.

Under certain circumstances there is a statutory requirement to consult with an advocate (IMCAs, 📖 Chapter 11), but there are many other occasions when having an experienced outsider to moderate between opposing factions can be of great benefit to the person with dementia and the care team in helping find a way forward. Health and social care authorities should employ independent advocates; if they don't it is often possible to find the appropriate person from the voluntary sector (e.g. Age Concern or the Alzheimer's Society).

Who should talk to whom?

If a patient is able to understand them, information and explanations should be directed at him or her. Decisions should be made by the person to whom they apply. Who else they want to be told, or to help or support them in making decisions (even a partner or children), is up to them. You should not get yourself in the position of telling relatives something that you have not told a patient who is in a position to be told.

An extreme view of confidentiality does not represent good practice either. Strictly, we should say nothing to anyone about a patient's health state except to the person themselves, unless they give permission. However, confidentiality has to be traded off against pragmatism and courtesy.

If a patient is severely ill, unable to understand, communicate, or otherwise speak for themselves, naturally close relatives will be concerned and want to know what is going on. Family members may be the only source of important information about someone's medical past and their likely wishes. Some have argued that the usual approach to ethics in dementia is inadequate, and a particular emphasis should be given to relationships, communication, and narrative (someone's previous experiences and life story). These ideas are particularly well expounded in the book *Ethical issues in dementia care: making difficult decisions* by Julian Hughes and Clive Baldwin (London: Jessica Kingsley, 2006).

If no family is available, do not forget other sources of useful information: GPs; district nurses; neighbours; wardens (of warden-aided flats); and social services. Watch out for visitors.

Taking the lead on decision-making has traditionally fallen to doctors, but there is no special reason why this should be so. Sometimes a problem can be introduced by one professional and followed up by another, e.g. if a difficult decision needs to be broken gently, if time is needed to think the problem through, or if others need to be consulted. Senior medical staff should be available and willing to support others in this role.

Summary

1. Consent must be gained for any examination, investigation, or treatment. It may be implicit or explicit, written or verbal. For consent to be valid, sufficient information must be given for a decision to be made.
2. Assume that someone is capable of giving consent unless you can show otherwise.
3. Capacity to consent requires that the person understands the proposed treatment, can retain and weigh up the information to come to a decision, and can communicate it.
4. If someone does not have capacity, act in their best interest. But first make sure you know what that best interest is, by asking people who might be able to provide the information you need.
5. If a decision is to be made, first consider feasibility—do the potential benefits outweigh the potential burdens? Then consider desirability—what does the patient want you to do, or what would the patient have wanted you to do?
6. Patients with dementia may or may not have capacity to consent.
7. Many people with severe dementia are approaching death. Best interest is not necessarily served by aggressive intervention, but it might be. The trick is to determine which, and this can be hard.

Measurement and rating scales

Introduction

Assessment scales are commonly used in dementia. Take care to use these tools for the right reasons, rather than as an exercise in measuring because it is possible. Poor selection and interpretation of data can prove a disservice to clients.

Dementia is an area where we often have to rely on informants other than the patient. In later stages of the illness the person with dementia may not be able to give an account of their symptoms and this can cause problems. In the 'grey' area of early presentations of cognitive impairment, the balance between self and proxy data gathering is most difficult to manage. With some dementia presentations insight may be impaired, in others the client may be psychologically defensive or avoidant, particularly if they have not sought referral in the first place. People with cognitive impairments understandably attempt to minimize the extent of their problems. Conversely, a desperate and worried carer may make great efforts to impress upon the assessing clinician the extent of the difficulties and provide an equally misleading picture (📖 Chapter 2). Good history takers are aware of these problems and balance the merits of different sources of information. The addition of objective measures can be very useful, as long as their psychometric properties (how good they are at measuring what they say they do) are well understood and their limitations taken into account. Numbers are reassuring but can mask the complexity of presentations and create a misleading picture of certainty and truth (📖 Chapter 2 p. 26).

How good is a rating scale?

All measures need to be assessed in a number of ways.

At what level are they measuring?

The level of measurement depends on the properties of the unit of measurement used. At their most basic these can be categorical (with no comparable quantity such as black and white) or continuous (with comparable properties such as higher and lower). Commonly used schemes include:

- Nominal: categorical properties such as yes/no or black/white, or different diagnoses.
- Ordinal: categories that can be put in order, e.g. from least to most, or best to worst.
- Interval: equal points between items such as temperature. For example the difference between 10°C and 11°C is the same as that between 12°C and 13°C.
- Ratio: equal points between items and a measure of zero. For example mass.

Make sure you know at what level measurement is taking place. For example many cognitive measures may give the impression of measuring at an interval or ratio level but may actually be ordinal in nature. Imagine a cognitive measure scored out of 50. Patient A scores 25 points at admission and 50 points at discharge. It can be tempting to say that they are twice as good at discharge as at admission. However, very few instruments have measurement properties that would justify this statement and it may be more accurate to say there has been an improvement that is clinically significant or statistically significant, provided the measure has properties that can support this.

Are they valid?

Does the measure capture the information that it claims to capture? For example an MMSE score of 10 out of 30 may indicate severe cognitive impairment. However, if a patient has problems with communication this may be very misleading.

Are they reliable?

Do they produce the same result on different occasions?

This depends on wording, understanding, and interpretation. Many assessment tools have a standardized format for administration. If this format is not followed it can jeopardize their reliability. All things being equal, a good measure should produce the same result on different occasions and with different raters. If it doesn't then we cannot trust the findings. More importantly, if we measure a change, then we need to be confident that this constitutes a real difference and not just the variation of different test administrations (e.g. different raters or improvement due to practice effects).

For the MMSE test-retest reliability is no better than +/- 4 points.

Are they sensitive?

If we are using the measure to detect something will it pick up the presence of that problem?

For example the MMSE will pick up cognitive impairment, but in higher functioning individuals it may not be sensitive enough to pick up that impairment until it is fairly advanced for that person.

Are they specific?

If the measure picks up a difference, is it the difference that we are interested in?

Sensitivity and specificity are frequently balanced against each other. For example a clock drawing task is very sensitive to dysfunction but has relatively low specificity regarding the cause of the problem.

Measures commonly used in clinical practice

The following sections review various questions and measurement strategies. There is no attempt to make this list exhaustive and readers may favour other instruments over those mentioned. We have tried to include those in most common usage. The aim is to increase awareness of the principles underpinning measurement and to encourage clinicians to make informed choices about measurement. As with any dynamic and developing area of clinical practice, new tools are appearing all the time.

Cognitive and neuropsychological assessment

The main principle underpinning the majority of these instruments is deficit measurement. This presupposes a normal or ideal level of functioning against which current performance can be measured. This can either be normative (derived from an appropriate population) or individual (from the patient's own history). In practice it is often a mixture of these two.

The scope of measurement in this area is immense and impossible to review comprehensively. In the light of this, tools have been divided into screening tools, tests of specific cognitive domains, and batteries.

Screening tools

The main characteristic of a screening tool is the imposition of a cut-off point. This is a point beyond which it is viewed that 'caseness' has been established. Statistical judgements are made by balancing sensitivity (can real cases be identified?) and specificity (are non-cases identified as normal?) for each measure and a point chosen beyond which it is assumed that the measured factor is present.

Cognition

Cognitive screening tools are widely used and have great clinical utility. (📖 Box 13.1). However, they should be interpreted with caution. The measurement of cognition covers a huge range of domains and screening tools may not allow comments to be made relating to specific areas of cognition. For example one crucial area of cognitive functioning such as frontal lobe functioning may catastrophically compromise many other areas, providing a misleading picture of overall cognition.

'**Box 13.1 Cognitive screening tools**

Clinical cognitive assessment in those with suspected dementia should include examination of attention and concentration, orientation, short- and long-term memory, praxis, language, and executive function. As part of this assessment, formal cognitive testing should be undertaken using a standardized instrument. The Mini-Mental State Examination (MMSE) has been frequently used for this purpose, but a number of alternatives are now available, such as the 6-item Cognitive Impairment Test (6-CIT), the General Practitioner Assessment of Cognition (GPCOG), and the 7-Minute Screen. Those interpreting the scores of such tests should take full account of other factors known to affect performance, including educational level, skills, prior level of functioning and attainment, language, and any sensory impairments, psychiatric illness, or physical/neurological problems.'

NICE Dementia Guideline p22 paragraph 1.4.1.3

Mini-Mental State Examination

This is probably the most widely used measure of cognition in clinical practice today. It is quick and easy to administer, provides a cut-off point, and divides scores into a number of different domains. It measures overall cognition and caution should be used when interpreting individual domains. It may also fail to measure deficits in highly capable individuals in the early stages of their illness. See also Chapter 2, p36.

Some notes of caution:

- Folstein's original MMSE used serial sevens and did not have the option of spelling WORLD backwards. It was this version that was used in the drug trials and that should be adopted when deciding on eligibility for AChEI.
- Don't always ask for the same three items for recall. People may benefit from a practice effect that was not intended in the original administration.
- MMSE scores will vary depending on where the test is done. It is much easier to be oriented at home than in a hospital.

Other tools

The following tools are also widely used (although this is not an exhaustive list):

- 6-item Cognitive Impairment Test (6-CIT).
- The General Practitioner Assessment of Cognition (GPCOG).
- The 7-Minute Screen.
- Abbreviated Mental Test (AMT).
- DemTect.
- Blessed Dementia Scale.
- Alzheimer's Disease Assessment Scale—Cognitive (ADAS-Cog) (used in all clinical trials but too complex for routine clinical practice).
- Clifton Assessment Procedure for the Elderly Cognitive Assessment Scale (CAPE-CAS).

- Brief Cognitive Rating Scale (BCRS).
- Large Allen Cognitive Level (LACL).
- Middlesex Elderly Assessment of Mental State (MEAMS).
- Addenbrooke's Cognitive Examination (ACE-R—Hodges—incorporates the MMSE but with wider domain coverage).

More details are given in Table 13.1.

Table 13.1 Examples of cognitive screening tools

Test name	Time (minutes)	Cost	Strengths/weaknesses
Mini-Mental State Examination http://www.minimental.com/	5	$130.00	Strengths: Quick and easy to administer. Good face validity. Covers a variety of domains. Weaknesses: Poor adherence to original standardization. Domain specificity is questionable. The location of testing can affect orientation scores.
6-item Cognitive Impairment Test (6-CIT) http://www.kingshill-research.org/kresearch/6cit.ASP	5	Free	Strengths: High sensitivity. Weaknesses: Scoring can be confusing.
7-minute Neurocognitive Screening Battery (7 min screen) http://www.memorydoc.org	7	Free	Strengths: Good test/retest reliability. Good sensitivity and specificity. Weaknesses: Scoring is confusing.
Abbreviated Mental Test http://www.racgp.org.au/silverbookonline/4-3.asp	5	Free	Strengths: Very simple to complete. Weaknesses: Very little validity data.
DemTect	5	Free	Strengths: Very simple to complete. Good specificity. Weaknesses: Specificity may compromise sensitivity.

Tests of specific cognitive domains

Tests of specific cognitive domains are most commonly administered by a neuropsychologist or other specialist. They usually form part of a wider selection of tests or follow a screening procedure that has generated questions about a specific aspect of cognitive functioning.

The following tests could be administered by any health or social professional:

Clock Drawing Test (praxis)

Draw a circle about 3 cm in diameter and mark the centre. Ask the patient to put in the numbers as they appear on a clock face. Then ask them to put in the hands to make it show ten past eleven. There are a number of schemes to score this test, but for most purposes it is possible to get an idea of whether there is dyspraxia (🕮 Figs. 13.1–4).

Word generation (Controlled Oral Word Association Test)

Ask the patient to list as many words as they can (excluding proper nouns) in one minute. This can be done using either words beginning with a particular letter of the alphabet (conventionally F, A, and S) or words from a particular category e.g. animals, flowers, or things you can eat. A normal score would be above 15 words/minute. Use several trials and take an average. There is some advantage in using categories as this allows you to assess the strategy they are using, e.g. for animals do they list farm animals or zoo animals together? (This tests verbal fluency and aspects of frontal lobe functioning.)

Trail-making Test (set shifting)

Draw numbers 1–10 randomly around a sheet of paper and ask the patient to draw a line from 1 to 2 to 3 etc. Measure the time. Repeat the test using numbers 1–5 and letters A–E, getting the patient to alternate between letters and numbers, i.e. 1–A, A–2, 2–B, B–3 etc. Patients with executive dysfunction have difficulty switching from letters to numbers. The first test is included to control for patients who have movement difficulties. Printed versions with norms are available.

Cognitive Estimates (grandiosity)

This consists of a number of questions that the patient is unlikely to know the correct answer to, but should be able to make a well informed guess. Patients with grandiosity give exaggerated responses. (Perry, R. and Hodges, J. R. 1999 *Brain*; **122**: 383–404.)

Note

Many of the above tests can be affected by problems in other domains (e.g. Clock Drawing is highly vulnerable to executive dysfunction). Using these tests in isolation can produce a misleading picture of the nature of cognitive impairment.

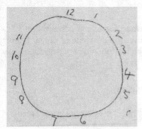

Fig. 13.1 August 1997 – First contact. Moderate impairment.

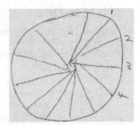

Fig. 13.2 December 1997 - AChEI started. More severe impairment.

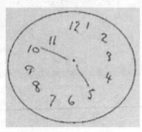

Fig. 13.3 February 1998. Good response after 2 months treatment.

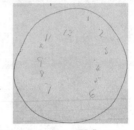

Fig. 13.4 October 1998. Response after 8 months.

Test batteries

Many batteries of tests have been developed for use in general and non-clinical populations. Their clinical use follows the principle of deficit testing and most require specific professional qualification and registration, usually as a neuropsychologist.

The most widely used batteries are:
- Wechsler Adults Intelligence Scale (WAIS-III).
- Wechsler Memory Scale (WMS-III).
- Repeatable Battery for the Assessment of Neuropsychological Status (RBANS).
- Cambridge Neuropsychological Test Automated Battery (CANTAB).
- Cambridge Examination for Mental Disorders of the Elderly revised (CAMDEX-R).

Measurement in other areas

Measurement in other areas

A variety of measures are in common usage looking at a number of areas. They employ a number of strategies including self report, checklists, informant report, and observation. Some employ specific cut-offs whilst others use the clinician's judgement.

NICE guidance recommends the use of the MMSE, together with global, functional, and behavioural assessments, in the monitoring of patients receiving AChEI (📖 Box 6.2). If specific tools are required for ADL or behavioural assessment we recommend the use of the Bristol ADL scale (📖 Box 13.2) and the NPI-Q (📖 Box 13.3).

Mood

- Geriatric Depression Scale.
- Cornell Scale for Depression in Dementia.
- Beck Depression Inventory.
- Hospital Anxiety and Depression Rating Scale.
- Beck Anxiety Inventory.
- Brief Assessment Schedule Depression Cards (BASDEC).

Activities of daily living

- Bristol Activities of Daily Living Scale (📖 Box 13.2).

Behaviour rating scales

- Neuropsychiatric Inventory (📖 Box 13.3).
- Behave-AD.
- Cohen-Mansfield Agitation Inventory.
- Challenging Behaviour Rating Scale.

Box 13.2 Bristol ADL scale

This scale rates 20 items from (a) to (e). The items include preparing and consuming food and drinks, dressing and personal hygiene, housework, mobility, communication etc.

For each activity, the rating indicates:
(a) performance unimpaired.
(b) mild impairment.
(c) moderate impairment.
(d) unable to perform task.
(e) not applicable.

Operational definitions are given for grades (a) to (d). The test takes about 15 minutes to complete on the basis of a carer interview. It is not copyright and requires no specific training.

Bucks et al. 1996 *Age and Ageing*; **25**: 113–20

Box 13.3 Neuropsychiatric Inventory

There are a number of published and validated variants of the NPI. The simplest is the NPI-Q, which is rated on the basis of an interview with a carer about the patient's behaviour during the past month. Twelve possible domains of behaviour that may cause problems are assessed:

- Delusions.
- Hallucinations.
- Agitation/Aggression.
- Depression/Dysphoria.
- Anxiety.
- Elation/Euphoria.
- Apathy/Indifference.
- Disinhibition.
- Irritability/Lability.
- Motor disturbance.
- Night-time behaviour.
- Appetite and eating.

If a symptom from a domain is present, it is graded on a three point scale of severity (1–3) and a six point scale (0–5) of distress to the carer. (The full NPI also includes a rating of frequency, 1–4).

In the clinical monitoring of patients the value of the scale is more as a checklist than as a formal rating procedure.

Carers

- Problem Checklist and Strain Scale.
- Ways of Coping Checklist.
- Screen for Caregiver Burden.
- Carer Strain Index.
- Burden Interview.
- Marital Intimacy Scale.
- Revised Memory and Behaviour Checklist.
- General Health Questionnaire (GHQ).

Dementia care mapping

This is a time sampling technique that is used to map care environments and the individual's experience and well-being (📖 Box 13.4).

Box 13.4 Dementia care mapping

Dementia Care Mapping (DCM) is designed to assess the quality of care from the perspective of the person with dementia. It was developed by Professor Tom Kitwood and Kathleen Bredin in the late 1980s. DCM uses a prescribed format for observing and recording staff and client interactions and then using this feedback to work with staff to facilitate change and improvements. It has been used in a variety of formal care settings including hospitals, care homes, and day care units. Training is required before this technique is used and is administered by the Bradford Dementia Group. The technique has its roots in person-centred care and the concept of personhood is of paramount importance (📖 Chapter 4 p. 78).

Quality of life measures
- DemQOL.

Global scales
- Clinical Dementia Rating (CDR).
- Global Deterioration Scale (GDS)—not to be confused with Geriatric Depression Scale.

Measures and measurement issues for specific populations

Drivers

Stroke Drivers Screening Assessment—although designed for use after stroke, this has been evaluated in dementia and seems to offer some guidance on likely hazardous driving. If a person with dementia wishes to continue driving and there are real concerns, then an on-road assessment at a specialized disabled drivers assessment centre is preferable.

Learning difficulties

This area covers a huge variety of presentations and judging progressive cognitive impairment can be difficult. However, there are some specific measures available (📖 Chapter 14).
- Neuropsychological Assessment of Dementia in Individuals with Intellectual Disabilities (NAID).
- Dementia Scale for Down's Syndrome (DSDS).

Black and minority ethnic populations

The cultural appropriateness of measures is a crucial issue here. Many tools will have been standardized against predominantly white Western populations, although commercial test developers are increasingly mindful of this problem and may include other population norms. Care must be taken if using tools in translation to ensure that revised norms are available or that the translated version has been properly validated. Care should also be taken if using existing tools via a translator as this may violate the assumptions of the original test.

As always, no assumptions should be made about individuals without a thorough assessment of their personal needs and cultural background having taken place.

Young people with dementia

Generally speaking cognitive tools have been standardized and normative data developed across the entire age range (although children and adults are commonly separated). If tools are specifically targeting older people then the manual should be consulted to ensure that they are validated against a younger population. Similarly many of the commercially available batteries do not extend beyond 89 years of age in their normative samples.

Educational issues

There will always be differences in the characteristics of different cohorts and test norms will have to be updated as different generations age. Many tests correlate highly with educational ability and opportunity. Even factors such as changes to school leaving age and the availability of free further and higher education can have an impact. Care should always be taken to be mindful of the general characteristics of different cohorts and also the age and applicability of any normative data.

Sources of rating scales

Most of the rating scales discussed in this chapter can be found online by entering their names in an internet search engine. One useful compendium (which also includes much else of value) is the Royal Australian College of General Practitioners 'Silver Book' on the medical care of older people in residential aged care facilities.

http://www.racgp.org.au/silverbookonline/index.asp

Many tests are included in: Burns, A., Lawlor, B., and Craig, S. 1999. *Assessment scales in old age psychiatry*. London: Martin Dunitz.

Strauss, E., Sherman, E. M. S., and Spreen, O. 2006. *A compendium of neuro-psychological tests: Administration, norms and commentary* (3rd edition) Oxford: OUP.

Summary

1. Dementia is a challenging area in which to apply standardized measures due to the nature of cognitive impairment and the characteristics of individual presentations.

2. There are a variety of measures that have great clinical utility.

3. However, care should always be taken to understand the properties and limitations of different measurement strategies so that results are not misinterpreted.

Chapter 14

Issues with particular groups of people

Dementia in people of working age

Epidemiology

Dementia is generally thought of as being a disease of older people, but it is commoner than most other neurological conditions in people of working age. Age-specific rates for dementia are shown in Table 14.1. Young onset dementia accounts for 2.2% of all people with dementia in the UK. There are at least 15 000 people with young onset dementia known to services in the United Kingdom (cf. nearly 700 000 people with onset after the age of 65 years). In a community of 250 000 people there are likely to be 100–150 people under 65 with dementia.

The causes of dementia in people under 65 are similar to those in older people, but with important differences. Alzheimer's disease and vascular dementia are the most common causes of dementia in people of working age, but the preponderance of Alzheimer's disease is less at only 30% of cases. Fronto-temporal and alcohol-related dementias are much more common and dementia with Lewy bodies is less frequent in this age group. A fifth of cases are associated with other neurological conditions, such as Huntington's disease and multiple sclerosis, which are rarely found in older people (or are hidden amongst the much larger numbers of people with the commoner dementias).

Table 14.1 Age-specific dementia rates

Age range/y	Rate/1000
30–39	0.1
40–49	0.2
50–54	0.5
55–59	1.5
60–64	2
65–69	15
70–74	35
75–79	60
80–84	125
85–89	200
90–94	300
95–99	350

Particular problems

'Younger people with dementia have special requirements, and specialist multidisciplinary services should be developed, allied to existing dementia services, to meet their needs for assessment, diagnosis, and care.' (NICE, 2006).

There are many features of young onset dementia that are different:
- Dementia in people under 65 is relatively rare, so it is less likely to be recognized. People with dementia and their carers have difficulty knowing where to turn for support; they may be referred to several different agencies for assistance with varying aspects of their problems.
- Younger people are more likely to have dependent children and still be working at the time of diagnosis. They will probably have to retire early and may not be immediately eligible for their full pension. Partners may have to give up work to care for the person with dementia and there are likely to be additional expenses in providing for dependent children. Family carers of younger people with dementia experience particular strain.
- Where services are designed primarily for older individuals, younger people may feel estranged and uncomfortable.
- The emotional impact of receiving a diagnosis of dementia will be greater and have a more dramatic effect on future plans. Needs for information and emotional support may be different for people of working age.
- The issues for younger people are likely to change more rapidly.

A survey of younger people with dementia in South West England revealed other issues as well (□ Box 14.1).

Box 14.1 Views of the specific needs of younger people with dementia compared with older people

- Physically fitter/more active.
- Appearance looks 'normal' (i.e. not like they have dementia).
- Have more energy.
- Need more social interaction.
- Less likely to get a speedy diagnosis.
- Their dementia is likely to progress more quickly.
- More likely to be working (along with their carers).
- More likely to be sexually active.
- More likely to have school age children.
- Family may resent intrusions by home care staff.
- Have more affinity with (younger) care staff than with (older) service users.
- Need a higher staff ratio and more activities.

Table 14.2 Common causes of dementia in people <65 (Harvey *et al.*, 2003)

Clinical diagnosis	Percentage
Alzheimer's dementia	35
Vascular dementia	20
Fronto-temporal	10
Alcohol	10
Dementia with Lewy bodies	5
Other	20

Table 14.3 Other causes of dementia in people <65 (Harvey *et al.*, 2003)

Disease	Rate/100 000
Huntington's disease	5
Multiple sclerosis	4
Down's syndrome	2
Cortico-basal degeneration	1
Prion disorders	1
AIDS dementia	1
Others	4
Total	18

JNNP (2003) 74 1206–9

Services for younger people with dementia

There are few cases of dementia in older people that are not due to AD, VaD, or DLB, but in younger people the causes are more varied (📖 Tables 14.2 and 14.3). It is helpful for younger people with dementia to be assessed by a neurologist. Unfortunately many neurologists have little interest in disorders of cognition. However, liaison psychiatrists, neuropsychiatrists, and general adult or old age psychiatrists who develop a special interest can all acquire the required expertise. Once the diagnosis is established, (all age) dementia services are generally best placed to provide continuing monitoring, help, and support.

Young people with dementia form a very heterogeneous group. Arranging an appropriate care package can be difficult. Many women of 64 years will fit well into services designed for older people with dementia, but younger men are generally not suited for older people's services. People with fronto-temporal dementia (📖 Chapter 15 p. 352) are especially difficult to accommodate, and with their activity, disinhibition, and hyperorality, often need one-to-one care. In addition, younger people with conditions such as MS and Huntington's disease may require specialist physical care.

Specialist services for younger people with dementia are best organized by developing an assembly of professionals (and volunteers) with skills in working with these problems. Whether they work together in one team or as sub-specialists in generic mental health teams will depend on local circumstances. Except in large conurbations, it is unlikely that there will be a sufficient number of people of working age with dementia to make specialist premises for day and residential care a viable proposition.

When planning new services it is best to start by designating a key person to start developing specialized resources (perhaps a social worker or CPN). Younger people with dementia themselves, and their carers, can make a valuable contribution to working out the best configurations of a service for a particular locality and should always be involved in the planning process. The Alzheimer's Society and other voluntary groups will also have valuable expertise. Early priorities in the development of specialized resources for younger people should include diagnostic facilities and community support. Arrangements for day care and respite care will also need to be considered (📖 Chapter 5 p. 118–120).

One of the great satisfactions of working with older people with dementia is the wealth of life experiences that they bring with them. Even if they are no longer able to take in new information, they are usually able to recall the era of their early lives in vivid detail. Developing forgetfulness in old age is not so unexpected, and providing behaviour is not too severely impaired, families often manage to cope well when one member becomes cognitively impaired.

By contrast it is immensely stressful working with younger people who have been deprived of experiencing the prime of their lives, whose children may miss out on expected parenting, and who may never have achieved financial security.

It is generally possible to share a diagnosis of dementia with an older person without causing undue distress to oneself or the person with dementia, but confirming that a young person has an irreversible and progressive brain disease is an emotionally draining experience for everyone involved.

Things can change fast for younger people and their families. Contact with services is especially important, as is knowing where to find help for problems that may affect almost any aspect of family life.

Dementia in people with learning disability

There are 1.4 million people with learning disability in England and this figure is growing. People with learning disability (LD) are at increased risk of developing dementia at a relatively young age. Staff working in the field of LD need special expertise to recognize early features of dementia. Health and social care professionals working in the field of dementia will encounter people with LD. There is a need for collaboration between LD and dementia services to share knowledge and experience. Both teams need to educate acute hospitals in the care of people with dementia. People with LD should not be excluded from any services because of their diagnosis, but care for people with LD is usually best provided by specialized LD teams.

People with LD sit on a spectrum of cognitive, functional, and behavioural ability. Most will be in one form or other of supported living arrangement, although some will live with (ageing) parents and others will be more or less independent. Dementia in people with LD is likely to present with deterioration from a previous level of functioning, in terms of memory, activities of daily living, behaviour, or psychological distress. Problems must be thoroughly assessed and understood. As with older people, physical factors and comorbidities must be excluded or taken into account. Changes to living or care arrangements, if any, must be made on the basis of assessed problems, and are likely to need review over time. However, for someone already in a highly supported environment, such as a residential home, apart from explaining why someone's abilities or mental health has changed, little extra may need to be done.

People with Down's syndrome are at risk of developing dementia from their forties, and the overall prevalence of dementia in people over 65 with LD from other causes is 2–3 times higher than in the general population. The pathological features of dementia in Down's syndrome are similar to those found in Alzheimer's disease, and there are similar neurochemical changes (◻ Chapter 16 p. 368) with reduction in acetylcholine, so treatment with cholinesterase inhibitors may be beneficial. Members of dementia teams may be able to share their experience of the practical issues associated with treatment with their LD colleagues (◻ Chapter 6 p. 140).

Brain scans (especially SPECT) may be abnormal in people with LD who do not have dementia, so the diagnosis needs to be made on the basis of the development of clinical features of dementia. However, physical illnesses and functional psychiatric disorders may produce similar changes in the functioning of people with LD, so comprehensive assessment by staff familiar with people with LD is essential.

The assessment needs to cover similar areas to those in any memory clinic (◻ Chapter 2 p. 30) but requires specialist expertise in the field of learning disability.

Assessment of cognitive impairment in people with LD

Physical assessment:
- Is there a physical disorder (particularly hypothyroidism or gastro-oesophageal reflux, but also epilepsy or cerebrovascular disease) that could be contributing?
- Problems with seeing, hearing, mobility?

Clinical history and mental state examination:
- Are there current social stresses—especially bereavement or other family issues?
- Are there comorbid psychiatric conditions—especially depression?

The history should be taken from an informant who has had knowledge of the person over time. It may be helpful to talk to more than one informant.

Neuropsychological assessment:
This should use measures specifically developed for dementia in people with LD. Where possible there should be a combination of direct and informant-based assessment. Possible tools include:
- Direct assessment of the individual:
  - British Picture Vocabulary Scale (BPVS).
- Informant-based assessment to address dementia-related changes and skills:
  - Dementia Questionnaire for Mentally Retarded Persons (DMR)
  - Gedye's Dementia Scale for Down's syndrome—this is not only appropriate for people with Down's syndrome (DSDS).

Occupational therapy assessment:
An OT should undertake a functional assessment to aid diagnosis and to monitor deterioration if relevant. NICE recommend the use of an Assessment of Motor and Process Skills should be used if treatment with an AChEI is proposed.

A case conference, bringing the specialists who have made assessments together, is helpful to formulate a diagnosis and plan management. This may include medical intervention, therapy or psychological intervention, and/or referral on to other disciplines (e.g. continence advice, dentistry, or vision services) depending on the problems. In every case social care arrangements, including those for living and personal care, will need to be reviewed.

Where there is uncertainty about the possibility of dementia, reassessments may need to be undertaken 12 or 24 months later. After 24 months, even if uncertainty remains, repeated assessment is not likely to be useful unless there is evidence that something has changed.

If a definite diagnosis of dementia is reached, treatment with an AChEI can be considered. NICE recommend using Dalton's Brief Praxis Test or the DMR for monitoring response to treatment.

Information on these tests can be found at the American Association on Intellectual and Developmental Disabilities at:
http://www.aamr.org/Reading_Room/Battery/battery_resources.pdf

Dementia in people from black and minority ethnic groups

Specific problems with dementia in people from ethnic minority groups have only recently been acknowledged as an issue. There is little research and few formal guidelines; the research that has been undertaken does not give any guidance as to how services should be developed.

First generation migrants are generally fit young people seeking political freedom or economic and social advancement. They leave behind the elderly and less fit members of the population. As migrants grow old themselves they may find themselves in an awkward position. Retaining ties to their homeland, they can become isolated from their children who have grown up in a different culture. Some second generation immigrants are unable to speak their parents' mother tongue. Isolation can be especially acute in people with dementia who lose their acculturation to their adopted country along with other aspects of their recent memory.

Migrants are as diverse as the countries from which they originate. Dementia occurs in people of all races. Studies in people of African and Asian origin in the USA have shown higher rates of dementia amongst African Americans in America than in areas from which they originated. Increased rates of dementia have been reported amongst people of Afro-Caribbean origin and also those from Greece and Turkey. Suggestions of a low rate of dementia amongst elderly Asians have not been confirmed. Indeed there are no recent epidemiological data on the prevalence of dementia in Asians in the UK. It is likely that vascular dementia is more common in Afro-Caribbean people and those from the Indian subcontinent, because of their increased prevalence of vascular risk factors. The frequency of the ApoE4 allele (📖 Chapter 16 p. 374) does appear to vary between ethnic groups but expression may be lower in Africans and Hispanic Americans.

One recent survey estimated that there are over 11 000 people from black and minority ethnic (BME) groups with dementia in the UK. 6.1% of working age (compared with 2.2% for the UK population as a whole). This suggests that either there is a particular susceptibility to pre-senile dementia amongst BME groups or a low prevalence of dementia amongst older BME people. In part this reflects the younger age profile of BME communities. There are relatively few very old members of these ethnic groups in the UK at present, but their numbers will grow as the population ages.

As well as the lack of any reliable data on the size of the problem, there are problems with using screening tools that were developed for use in white British and American people who have received formal education. The MMSE has been translated into Gujarati, Hindi, and Chinese but caution is needed in interpreting scores. A Hindi version developed for use in a UK population may not be valid in a person who has recently arrived from rural India.

Surveys in ethnic minority groups suggest that there may be problems of a lack of awareness of dementia, although there are comparable levels of ignorance about dementia in the indigenous population. Ethnic groups may be more inclined to rely upon informal family care rather than statutory services; it is not clear whether this is a result of cultural preferences or the inadequacy of formal arrangements. Elders from minority groups may put pressure on members of their families to provide care themselves rather than involve other agencies.

Assessing cognition is crucially dependent on adequate understanding and communication. If someone is not a fluent and confident English speaker, or has lost the ability to use English, adequate translation is an absolute pre-requisite for performing a meaningful assessment. If it is possible to identify a trusted professional colleague who understands the person's personal circumstances and who can convey what they are trying to express and explain what the care team are trying to do, this will generally be the best solution. Sometimes translators will go beyond simply translating words, and if suitably trained can translate ideas, or become a more general advocate or go-between. This can be immensely useful, so long as you know what is happening and exactly who is saying what.

A family member may be able to help, and will often be conveniently and immediately available. But this is not always without problems and hidden family tensions may be missed. Sometimes a 'conference call' (three-way telephone conversation, preferably using a speakerphone) can be arranged to translate, so long as the person with dementia is not too bewildered by the experience. Many hospitals keep registers of their staff with fluent second languages who can help, and with an increasingly mobile international workforce, very many languages can be available. Be careful; the fact that the translator works in a health or social care setting is not a guarantee that they will be sensitive and aware of cultural issues.

There are further catches for the unwary. Written materials in foreign languages may be of little benefit, as many people in Britain who cannot understand spoken English are not able to read their native language.

A professional translator may have to be used. These may be excellent but there may be clashes between different cultural groups from the same area, which are not acknowledged by agencies offering interpreters.

Neither practice nor academic research has offered any clear guidance as to whether it is better to provide mainstream services that are capable of addressing the needs of all ethnic and cultural groups, or to set up specialist services for a specific group. Once again it will be necessary to consider the needs of a particular locality and members of the local community. Many people of foreign origins identify closely with the host community and may wish to avoid being stereotyped as members of a minority group.

Specific needs of minority groups

Apart from issues around religion and language, people from ethnic minorities are likely to have preferences for bathing, skin care, hair care and diet which differ from those of the indigenous population. It is difficult to be specific about what these needs are for particular groups. Members of community teams can play a valuable educational role by increasing awareness of dementia and related issues with community leaders.

Adhering to the principles of person-centred care for all people with dementia will encompass the special requirements of people from BME backgrounds. As a general rule, minority ethnic groups are broad and open-minded, and if a modicum of sympathy for their particular situation is shown, satisfactory solutions to problems can be negotiated, as well as they can for indigenous populations (or, at least, they may be no more difficult than for indigenous populations!).

Potential problem areas
- Diet—vegetarian, Halal, kosher, other dietary taboos.
- Gender of carers—both men and women may find receiving care from a member of the opposite sex unacceptable.
- Toileting.
- 'Precedence' for elders within families.
- Elders who face a crisis whilst away from home (e.g. on holiday from Pakistan).

Summary

1. Dementia in younger people is not a rare disorder, but the causes and problems are different from those in older people.
2. People with learning disability are at increased risk of dementia, and special measures are required to diagnose and monitor dementia in this group of people.
3. Little work has been done on the specific problems faced by people with dementia from minority ethnic groups and their carers.

Rarer causes of dementia

Fronto-temporal dementia

Fronto-temporal dementia (FTD) is not common, particularly amongst older people. The term Pick's disease was formerly used for this condition. Although convenient—families find the term fronto-temporal dementia clumsy and difficult—the pathology described by Pick (🕮 Chapter 16) is actually only found in a minority of cases. They are relatively frequent in younger people with dementia, responsible for around 20% of dementia in people under 65 (second only to Alzheimer's disease).

The problem posed by people with FTD to their families is enormous. They also provide a great challenge to service providers, as their needs are very different from other people with dementia.

Symptoms

Like most other forms of dementia, FTD has an insidious onset and gradual progression (🕮 Box 15.1). Unlike other dementias the presenting symptoms are usually either abnormal behaviour or language disturbance. Personality changes are often prominent, with a loss of concern about social contact and disregard of conventions. People with FTD may become coarser in their language, drink excessively, and display aggression and hyperactivity. They lose insight into these changes in the early stages.

Language changes may be either a difficulty in finding words or being excessively verbose; in the later stages perseveration and echolalia are characteristic. On neurological examination primitive reflexes may be elicited or signs of stiffness and tremor.

Memory impairment may only occur late in the course of the disorder.

Patterns of FTD

A number of pathological processes may cause FTD (🕮 Box 15.2). The clinical picture is dependent on the site of the lesions, not their histology.

Motor neuron disease (MND)

Dementia associated with MND is the least uncommon cause of FTD in older people. It is different from other types of FTD—it is rapidly progressive and causes serious physical disability. FTD from other causes progresses slowly over a number of years, but MND dementia typically causes death within 1–2 years of the onset of symptoms.

About 20% of patients with MND develop overt psychological symptoms, although SPECT scanning and neuropsychological testing of people with MND reveal sub-clinical FTD in many more.

It may occur with both common types of motor neuron disease: progressive bulbar palsy and amyotrophic lateral sclerosis.

Box 15.1 Features of FTD

Core features

- Insidious onset and gradual progression.
- Early decline in social interpersonal contact.
- Early impairment in regulation of personal conduct.
- Early emotional blunting.
- Early loss of insight.

Supportive features

- Behaviour problems:
  - decline in personal hygiene and appearance
  - stubbornness
  - distractibility and impersistence
  - hyperorality and dietary changes
  - perseverative and stereotyped behaviour (repeatedly performing actions, such as checking an appliance is turned off, always in the same way)
  - utilization behaviour (difficulty resisting their impulse to 'utilize' objects that are in their visual field and within reach).
- Speech and language:
  - altered speech output (economy and aspontaneity of speech)
  - pressure of speech
  - stereotypy of speech
  - echolalia
  - perseveration
  - mutism.
- Physical signs:
  - primitive reflexes
  - incontinence
  - akinesia, rigidity, and tremor
  - low and labile blood pressure.

Box 15.2 Pathological causes of FTD

- Motor neuron disease.
- Non-specific atrophy and gliosis.
- Tauopathy (FTDP-17 and Pick's disease), see Chapter 16, p374.
- Neurofilamentopathy.

Progressive aphasia

In this condition the first symptom is usually difficulty finding words, although sometimes problems producing sound come first. As the disorder progresses, reading, writing, and other forms of language are also affected. After several years behaviour and cognitive changes also appear and in the final stages there is global cognitive impairment.

Semantic dementia

People with this condition are initially unable to remember connections between words and their meanings; other memories are less affected and episodic memory is typically preserved. There is slow progression to global dementia.

Behaviour and personality changes in FTD

This is a notoriously difficult condition to diagnose; the onset is insidious and the early symptoms are non-specific. Two types are recognized:

1. Overactive, disinhibited type:
   - Embarrassing behaviour in public, shouting, swearing, sexual talk (rarely any more than talk), overspending, wandering, stealing. Lack of insight into the effect their behaviour is having on other people.
   - Repetitive and stereotyped behaviour as the disorder progresses, e.g. repeatedly writing the same words or taking the same walk.

2. Apathetic and resistive type:
   - Loss of interest and motivation:
     - initially in hobbies and activities
     - later all activities of daily living, resisting attempts to maintain personal hygiene.
   - Excessive eating and indiscriminately putting objects in the mouth.

Investigation in FTD

The key investigation in suspected FTD is detailed neuropsychological testing. Impairment in verbal fluency and set shifting (e.g. on the trail making test), and grandiosity (cognitive estimates) (📖 Chapter 13) are pointers to the need for neuropsychological referral.

Physical investigation including MRI imaging is often normal even after gross language or behaviour changes are present. Serial scans may show evolving atrophy in the frontal or temporal areas, which may be unilateral. The EEG is invariably normal and laboratory tests are unhelpful. Genetic causes of FTD are relatively common—it is worth taking a detailed family history, and genetic counselling may be indicated.

Management

It is extremely difficult to help people with FTD or their families. With their behaviour and personality changes they do not easily adapt to care settings designed for people with Alzheimer's disease, and as the condition is uncommon there are very few specialized resources available. The principles of person-centred care are applicable (📖 Chapter 4) and the Pick's Disease Support Group (www.pdsg.org.uk) can offer guidance and counselling to families. There is no specific drug treatment, and medication for behaviour disturbance is of limited benefit.

Demyelinating disorders (MS and related conditions)

Cognitive impairment is common in people with multiple sclerosis (MS), particularly those with chronic progressive disease. 50–70% of MS patients have some degree of cognitive difficulties, most commonly problems with short-term memory and problem solving; this may occur in quite young people.

Verbal skills are often well-preserved. Depression is common in people with MS; the often-described 'euphoria' of MS is almost always associated with significant cognitive impairment.

Post-mortem studies have shown that MS dementia is associated with loss of acetylcholine and choline acetyltransferase, providing some evidence to support the use cholinesterase inhibitors in MS.

Huntington's disease

Huntington's disease is the commonest form of inherited dementia. The prevalence varies in different countries, but in North America and Western Europe is 4–8 cases/100 000 population.

It is caused by the accumulation of nonsense DNA on chromosome 4. The disorder is inherited as an autosomal dominant condition, showing genetic anticipation (with succeeding generations the symptoms start at an earlier age). It is also more virulent when inherited via the father.

Presenting symptoms of Huntington's vary depending on the age at first presentation, which can be anything between adolescence and old age. Symptoms in older people are more likely to be physical:
- Gait disturbance.
- Abnormal movements (choreiform).
- Little in the way of cognitive symptoms in the early stages.
- Less likely to be a clear-cut family history.

In those with earlier onset psychiatric symptoms are more prominent:
- Depression.
- Psychosis:
  - delusional mood
  - schizophrenia-like auditory hallucinations.
- Personality change.
- Behaviour disturbance:
  - aggression
  - hostility
  - loss of social control.

Early cognitive changes also occur in younger people:
- Slowness of response.
- Problems with serial arithmetic.
- Difficulty in switching between tasks.
- Impaired verbal fluency.
- Visuo-spatial problems.

Later global cognitive decline occurs, although insight may be preserved for some time.

Findings on brain imaging include dilated ventricles with more marked frontal lobe atrophy. SPECT may reveal diminished metabolism in the basal ganglia. The diagnosis can be established by molecular genetic studies. Once the diagnosis is clear it is important to refer family members for genetic counselling.

Progressive supranuclear palsy (PSP)

The key symptoms of PSP are paralysis of eye movements (especially difficulties in looking upwards), muscular rigidity, and cognitive impairment. Patients tend to adopt a hyperextended posture and often fall over backwards. The mental state is characteristic; people with PSP often have pronounced psychomotor retardation, but if given long enough can respond correctly. There may be changes in mood and behaviour, which may take the form of apathy and withdrawal or irritability and excitement; emotional lability is common. There is no specific treatment.

Prion disorders

Prions are proteins that can accumulate in the brain and cause dementia and other neurological disturbance.

Creutzfeldt-Jakob disease (CJD)

Classical CJD occurs in people between the ages of 45 and 75, mostly 60–65. After a period of vague ill health they develop rapidly progressive dementia, usually with myoclonus and other neurological signs such as ataxia, Parkinsonism, and cortical blindness. Most cases progress to death within 6 months. There are no specific features on MRI scanning. The EEG may show abnormal triphasic waves. In the UK, suspected cases should be referred to the CJD Surveillance Unit in Edinburgh.

Variant CJD (vCJD) was first described in the 1990s. It is thought to be due to infection by the agent responsible for bovine spongiform encephalopathy (BSE). It occurs in younger people (20–40 years).

Presenting features are often psychiatric:
• Anxiety.
• Depression.
• Schizophrenia—with typical hallucinations or delusions.
Later:
• Focal neurological signs.
• Cerebellar ataxia.
• Dementia.

The progression is slower than in classical CJD, with a median survival of 14 months. EEG features of classical CJD are not found, but there may be distinctive MRI changes in the thalamus.

There are genetic cases of CJD. The disorder may also be transmitted by the inoculation of infected material during medical procedures such as injection of human pituitary extract or the use of contaminated neurosurgical instruments.

Other prion disorders include Gerstmann-Straussler-Scheinker syndrome and fatal familial insomnia.

HIV-associated dementia

HIV infection is associated with a variety of cognitive impairments
(📖 Chapter 3 p. 67).

HIV-associated dementia (HAD, also called AIDS-dementia complex)
has insidious onset over months and is indistinguishable clinically from
other types of dementia, including forgetfulness, poor concentration, slowness, apathy, dyspraxia, and language problems. It is commoner in older
patients and those with more advanced disease. There is often associated
poor balance, clumsiness, and generalized weakness. Neurological signs
may be absent at first, but later include primitive reflexes, tremor, hyper-
reflexia, increased tone, and muscle weakness. Ultimately it progresses
(over months to years) to an end stage with severe mute dementia and
immobility.

Treatment with highly active anti-retroviral therapy (HAART) has
reduced the incidence of HAD (to about 10/1000 person years at risk)
and at least partially reverses established cognitive impairment. It has also
improved survival, which paradoxically has increased prevalence. However,
HAD can also develop during treatment with HAART, and treatment
failure is associated with rapidly worsening cognition. A minimally disabling
variant, called minor cognitive motor disorder (MCMD) is commoner than
established dementia (30% of HIV infected adults have MCMD compared
with 10% with dementia). In time, MCMD will progress.

Investigations include MRI scan (Fig. 15.1 and the Plate section)—patchy
or confluent periventricular white matter hyperintensity on T2 weighted
images (also to exclude tumours). Lumbar puncture reveals increased
protein in 60% and mononuclear cells in 25% (also excludes other infections). HIV and anti-HIV antibodies may be detected in CSF. Blood inflammatory markers are raised.

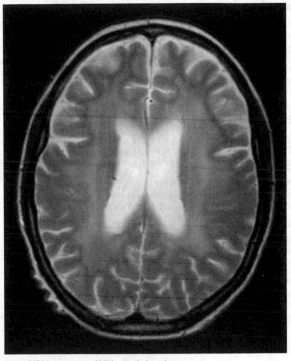

Fig. 15.1 MRI appearance of HIV encephalopathy.

Cortico-basal degeneration (CBD)

This rare disorder is unlikely to present initially to a memory clinic. It has some features of PSP and FTD. The initial symptoms are of unilateral rigidity, progressing to myoclonus and dyspraxia. 'Alien hand' (believing that one's hand is not one's own) is a characteristic symptom. Cognitive problems may be absent. About one-third of cases progress to global dementia.

Neurosyphilis

Syphilis occurs as a result of infection with the spirochaete *Treponema pallidum*, Neurosyphillis is not normally seen now except in people with syphillis and AIDS. There are two main patterns:

Meningovascular syphillis

This usually presents with recurrent strokes. Symptoms include diplopia (double vision), vertigo ataxia and dysarthria (slurring of speech).

General paralysis of the insane (GPI)

This condition classically presents with grandiose delusions, confabulation and personality change. There may be features of spinal cord involvement, producing loss of sensation in the feet and lightning pains.

Investigation

Serological blood tests for syphilis are the initial screen. If these are positive, refer to a genitourinary medicine clinic for definitive testing by lumbar puncture and further management, including contact tracing. People from Africa and the Caribbean may be liable to other treponemal infections which may produce false positive results on tests for syphilis.

Summary

1. Fronto-temporal dementia is a difficult condition to diagnose and treat. It most commonly occurs in association with motor neuron disease.
2. Many rarer causes of dementia are due to genetic factors. Counselling for family members should always be considered.
3. Close working relationships between neurologists and community health teams can help support people with disorders that cause problems with mobility and cognition.

Biological aspects of dementia

The ageing brain

Humans are unique in the extent to which the brain changes with age. The process of normal ageing causes changes in appearance that are very similar to those found in Alzheimer's disease, and there is a considerable overlap between the findings in healthy brains and those from people with dementia. Apart from a few reports in other higher primates such as chimpanzees these appearances have never been found in other species.

Structure

Macroscopic changes

- Shrinkage of the brain is normal with increasing age.
- The cerebral ventricles become dilated.
- Convolutions on the surface of the brain (gyri) become atrophied.
- This causes widening of the fissures between the gyri (sulci).
- The occipital lobes only show minor atrophy.
- Frontal lobes have some atrophy as part of normal ageing.
- The earliest signs of atrophy in Alzheimer's disease occur in the medial temporal lobe, which can be detected on MRI. MRI is the procedure of choice in the investigation of early Alzheimer's disease, particularly in younger people.
- The medial temporal lobe is important in laying down new memories, hence the earliest symptom in Alzheimer's disease is usually forgetfulness.
- Later in the course of the disease, younger people with Alzheimer's disease (those under about 75 years at onset) also develop more pronounced atrophy of the frontal and parietal lobes (◫ Fig. 16.1).
- Frontal lobe damage causes problems with executive functioning and verbal fluency.
- The parietal lobes are important in skilled motor activity (praxis).
- People with dementia developing in very late life (over 80) have only the temporal lobe showing significant shrinkage at post-mortem when compared against age matched control subjects.

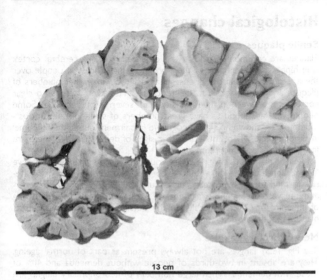

Fig. 16.1 Composite plate showing section through brain of a case of severe Alzheimer's Disease (left) and normal control (right). See also Plate 3, Plate section.

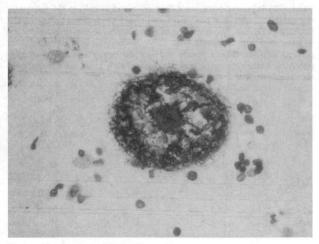

Fig. 16.2 Neuritic plaque. See also Plate 4, Plate section.

Histological changes

Senile plaques

Plaques are commonly found in the oldest part of the cerebral cortex (the hippocampus) as part of the normal ageing process in people over the age of 50. Alzheimer's disease is associated with higher numbers of plaques and with plaques in the neocortex. However, there is no clear correlation between plaque density and severity of dementia. Some people who are found to have great numbers of senile plaques at post-mortem have shown no sign of cognitive impairment during their lifetime; in other people where there are clear signs of dementia in life, there are few plaques at post-mortem.

Neuritic plaques (Fig. 16.2) are roughly spherical in shape. They have 'target' appearance, with a central core of extracellular amyloid material, formed from Aβ protein. This is surrounded by a zone of degenerating nerve cell elements, fragments of axons and dendrites, with a ring of inflammatory microglial cells on the outside. 'Primitive' or 'immature' plaques lack the amyloid core.

Neurofibrillary tangles

(Fig. 16.3) Tangles are not always present as part of normal ageing. They are absent in two-thirds of people without dementia and 40% of those with dementia. When large numbers of neurofibrillary tangles are present in the cortex, dementia is invariable.

Lewy bodies

(Fig. 16.4) Lewy bodies were first observed in cells in the substantia nigra and basal ganglia in post-mortem tissue from patients suffering from Parkinson's disease. The presence of Lewy bodies in the cerebral cortex is associated with dementia with Lewy bodies (DLB). Compared with patients with Alzheimer's disease and vascular dementia, cerebral atrophy only occurs late in the course of the disease; early brain scans may appear remarkably normal.

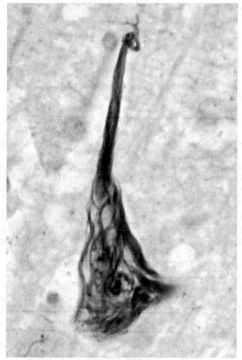

Fig. 16.3 Neurofibrillary Tangle. See also Plate 5, Plate section.

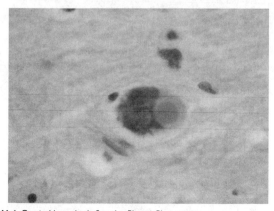

Fig. 16.4 Cortical Lewy body. See also Plate 6, Plate section.

Pick bodies

(📖 Fig. 16.5) In some cases of fronto-temporal dementia (Pick's disease), cells are found with distinctive inclusion bodies (Pick bodies) that cause swelling of the nerve cell body and compression of the nucleus.

Vascular changes

Large vessel disease

If cerebral blood vessels are blocked by blood clots that have formed *in situ* (thrombi) or that have been carried to the brain in the circulation (emboli), then regions of the brain will be deprived of oxygen and nutrients leading to cell death (infarction). This may cause the clinical signs of a stroke, but sometimes there are no symptoms. These areas of infarction may be visible on brain scans. Small areas of infarction are sometimes referred to as lacunes (📖 Fig. 16.6).

Dementia may result either from a single large infarct or from an accumulation of damage from multiple smaller infarcts. There are a few regions of the brain (such as the angular gyrus) where a single strategically placed infarct may cause dementia.

Small vessel disease

Blood vessels become less elastic with age as a result of fatty substances being deposited in their walls. This process is known as arteriosclerosis (📖 Fig. 16.6), 'hardening of the arteries'. It may lead to impaired circulation and a greater liability to strokes. Areas affected by this impaired circulation, especially around the cerebral ventricles, are known as leukoariosis.

Both large and small vessel disease is more common in people with dementia, although either may be present in people without dementia. Raised blood pressure, cholesterol, smoking, and diabetes accelerate the development of cerebrovascular disease.

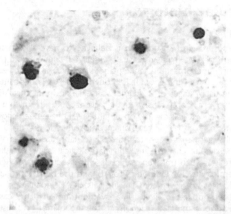

Fig. 16.5 Pick bodies stained to demonstrate τ protein. See also Plate 7, Plate section.

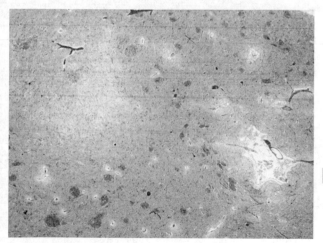

Fig. 16.6 Vascular dementia showing lacunar infarct (left) and arteriosclerosis (right). See also Plate 8, Plate section.

Molecular biology

Amyloid

Beta amyloid protein (Aβ or βA4) is believed to have a key role in the development of Alzheimer's disease. It is derived from amyloid precursor protein (APP). It is present in senile plaques in cerebral blood vessels and may be deposited in the brain. It is thought that Aβ is deposited in the brain in the early stages of Alzheimer's disease and that this Aβ is itself toxic to the brain and causes further damage ('the amyloid cascade hypothesis'). A few cases of early onset familial AD have been shown to be due to mutations of the APP gene on chromosome 21.

The faulty gene has been transferred to laboratory animals, which develop behaviour changes and the pathological signs of Alzheimer's disease. Treating such transgenic animals with inoculation of Aβ protein causes them to develop antibodies to Aβ, and the behavioural and pathological changes are reversed. Clinical trials of Aβ inoculation in people with AD have not led to clinical improvement, but in some cases there have been serious and fatal reactions to the inoculation. In these individuals senile plaques are not found in the brain, but there are signs of spaces (vacuoles) where it is believed that plaques were formerly situated.

Tau

Neurofibrillary tangles are derived from τ protein that has undergone an abnormal degree of phosphorylation. This causes the proteins to condense into paired helical filaments. τ protein normally forms part of the nerve cells' internal transport mechanism. Attempts to treat dementia by inhibiting the phosphorylation of τ protein have not been successful so far. τ protein abnormalities are also found in FTD, PSP, and CBD (□ Chapter 15).

Alpha-synuclein

α-synuclein is a protein that is found in Lewy bodies. It is normally present in synaptic vesicles. It is believed to play a role in the metabolism of neurofilaments.

Genetics of dementia

Global dementias

ApoE

Apolipoprotein E is a constituent of lipoproteins, whose function is to transport fats in the bloodstream. There are three forms of ApoE: ε2, ε3, and ε4. ε3 is the most common form, ε2 is relatively rare, and ε4 is the second most common. Many studies have shown that people carrying the ε4 allele have a higher risk of developing Alzheimer's disease, whilst ε2 is associated with a lower risk of having AD. The risk is highest in people carrying two ε4 alleles (ε4 homozygotes).

Single gene disorders

1. APP

The first confirmed genetic cause of Alzheimer's disease was a mutation of the amyloid precursor protein gene (see previous section) on chromosome 21. This genetic abnormality is a very rare cause of AD even amongst pedigrees where familial AD has been identified. A number of different loci on this gene may cause familial AD, but other mutations on nearby base pairs can cause hereditary cerebrovascular disease.

2. Presenilins

Mutations on the presenilin-1 gene (on chromosome 14) are the commonest cause of early onset familial AD. Many different mutations of these genes have been described, making screening tests to detect these changes very difficult. Affected individuals in these families display signs of cognitive impairment at a very young age (35–55 years). There is also a very similar gene (known as presenilin-2) on chromosome 1. Many fewer pedigrees have been reported for this gene, and the onset of illness is later in them. The physiological role of presenilin is not known.

3. α-synuclein (see previous section)

There are two recognized mutations of the gene for this protein, SNCA and SNCB, both of which are inherited in an autosomal dominant manner. The former causes Parkinson's disease, the latter dementia with Lewy bodies.

4. CADASIL

(Cerebral autosomal dominant arteriopathy with subcortical ischaemic changes and leukoencephalopathy). This is an inherited vascular dementia that occurs as a result of mutations on the NOTCH 3 gene on chromosome 19.

Fronto-temporal dementia

Tauopathy

Some cases of fronto-temporal dementia run in families. In many of these people there are signs of Parkinson's disease. The condition is known as fronto-temporal dementia with Parkinsonism (FTDP) and has been found to be associated with mutations in the gene for τ protein on chromosome 17.

Neurofilamentopathy

There are other structures apart from neurotubules present in nerve cell processes, known as neurofilaments. Abnormalities of neurofilament protein are an even rarer genetic cause of FTD.

SOD

About 10% of cases of motor neuron disease follow a familial pattern; about 15% of these are due to mutations of the SOD-1 gene for super-oxide dismutase, an enzyme that acts to quench free radicals in the brain.

Other genetic causes of dementia

Many other genetic causes of dementia, including a number of causes of vascular dementia, have been described, but they are all extremely rare.

Summary

1. The pathological changes of Alzheimer's disease are similar to those that occur with normal ageing, but are much more pronounced in dementia.
2. Specific biological markers can be found in dementia of other causes.
3. Understanding the biological basis of dementia may produce more effective treatments for dementia in the future.

Prevention

Why prevent?

'It is better to be healthy than to be ill or dead. That is the beginning and the end of the only real argument for preventive medicine. It is sufficient.' (Rose, 1992)

The idea of prevention is attractive, but preventative interventions must still be judged by the same criteria as any others. They must be effective, affordable, acceptable, humane, accessible, and equitable. Indeed, if the target population is more or less healthy, evaluation should be even more stringent than usual. The costs of prevention in terms of side effects, resources, time, inconvenience, and changes to lifestyle must be carefully weighed against likely benefits.

Four strands of evidence suggest whether a disease or condition is preventable:

- Variation in time and place, both between and within countries.
- Observations of migrants adopting the risk of their host environment.
- Whether risk varies according to personal characteristics, such as nutrition, toxic exposure, blood pressure, smoking, trauma history, and physical activity.
- Experimental evidence from randomized controlled trials demonstrating whether incidence reduces following interventions (e.g. vitamin supplementation or blood pressure reduction).

The observational epidemiology of dementia is less well worked out than for many other diseases, and there is little to suggest that Alzheimer's disease, dementia with Lewy bodies, or frontal type dementia can be prevented. The epidemiology of cerebrovascular disease is well worked out and prevention strategies well established.

Strictly, prevention means forestalling of the onset of a disease process or consequence. Closely related is screening or case finding, where early disease is systematically sought out to allow earlier intervention.

Preventing what?

Just considering prevention of pathology is unduly narrow. We might think of prevention at several further levels:

- Diseases or syndromes:
  - dementia
  - delirium (📖 Chapter 3 p. 70).
- Comorbidities:
  - falls, osteoporosis, vascular disease, infections.
- Complications:
  - pressure sores
  - fractures.
- Disability, distress, and dependency:
  - behavioural disturbance
  - activities of daily living
  - loss of 'personhood'
  - institutionalization
  - morbidity in carers.

Table 17.1a Risk factors for dementia and potential preventative strategies: non-modifiable factors

Risk factor	Effect
Age	Alzheimer's prevalence doubles every 4.5 years after 65. Possibly no increase after 50–60% prevalence in mid 90s.
Learning disability	Down's patients develop dementia 30–40 years early. Non-Down's learning disabled people have 2–3 times higher risk than general population.
Gender	Risk of AD is higher in women, risk of vascular dementia is higher in men.
Genes	<1% of all AD is familial; typically onset <55 years. Overall, perhaps 50% of AD risk is genetic.
Apolipoprotein E4	Risk for vascular and DLB. >50% of AD occurs in people without the apo ε4 allele.

Table 17.1b Risk factors for dementia and potential preventative strategies: modifiable factors

Risk factor	Effect
Cholesterol	Some (but not all) studies suggest hypercholesterolaemia is a risk for both vascular and Alzheimer's dementia. Cross-sectional studies suggest statin use is beneficial, but this has not been confirmed in trials, even where reduction in stroke and heart disease has been demonstrated. 📖 Box 17.1.
Antioxidants	Some evidence for a protective effect of vitamin E, but randomized trials (up to 5 years) so far disappointing. 📖 Box 17.1.
Blood pressure	Midlife hypertension is a risk for both vascular and Alzheimer's dementia. Meta-analysis of intervention studies shows a non-significant benefit for BP reduction. Regardless, abundant evidence indicates the value of treating high blood pressure to reduce strokes and heart disease. 📖 Box 17.2.
NSAIDs	Some studies show reduced dementia incidence with NSAIDs use. A meta-analysis was negative, although a moderate effect could not be excluded (summary relative risk 1.23, 95% CI 0.70–2.3). Clinical trials of flurbiprofen in cognitive impairment are in progress. 📖 Box 17.3.
Alcohol	Alcohol is neurotoxic and heavy drinkers risk thiamine deficiency and head injury. However, abstinence and excess both increase risks epidemiologically. Alcohol intake in recommended range is unlikely to increase risk. 📖 Box 17.4.
Smoking	Increased risk in longitudinal studies. 📖 Box 17.5.
HRT	Retrospective studies of women receiving HRT suggested it was protective against dementia, but randomized trials showed the opposite. 📖 Box 17.6.
Obesity	Dementia increased with midlife high body mass index, possibly secondary to diabetes.
Head injuries	Head injury sufficiently severe to produce loss of consciousness doubles the risk of dementia developing.

Homocysteine	Reduced intake of folate causes a rise in plasma homocysteine, which is associated with an increased risk of heart and cerebrovascular disease, including dementia. Preliminary evidence suggests increasing intake of folate slows decline in some cognitive tasks. □ Box 17.7.
Depression	Approximate doubling of the risk of dementia in people with a history of depression. Even a single episode of depression occurring 25 years before the onset of cognitive symptoms produces a measurable effect. The effect of treatment for depression is unknown.
Exercise	Midlife moderate exercise (30 minutes twice a week) halves risk of dementia in prospective studies, but there are no trials.
Education and mental stimulation	Low education appears to be a risk factor for dementia, but direct causation is uncertain. Some evidence suggests that regular, cognitively-stimulating activities reduce risk of dementia over 5 years or so, but interpreting whether this is a true protective effect is difficult.

Modified from: National Collaborating Centre for Mental Health. Dementia: supporting people with dementia and their carers in health and social care. 2006; National Clinical Practice Guideline No. 42. London; NICE. http://guidance.nice.org.uk/cg42

Prevention of dementia

Alzheimer's, DLB, and frontal type dementia

In practical terms there are no established, effective preventative interventions. Stopping smoking, reducing blood pressure, and moderating heavy alcohol intake may help, but are indicated regardless of their effects on dementia.

Vascular dementia

The presumed pathogenesis is the cumulative effects of multiple small infarcts. 10–20% of stroke survivors have cognitive impairment, which, while often patchy and non-progressive, in many ways resembles dementia. Preventing strokes therefore should prevent cognitive impairment (Table 17.2).

- Vascular prevention is very well researched, and a battery of interventions is generally offered to those who have suffered a heart attack, stroke, or peripheral vascular disease, or who are at high risk (2–3% per year) on the basis of age and vascular risk factors (blood pressure, cholesterol, diabetes, smoking). The empirical evidence for vascular prevention preserving cognitive function is weak.
- Subject to agreement and safe medicines management, it would be logical to offer standard vascular secondary prevention to people with vascular dementia. This might include 75 mg of aspirin (with a proton pump inhibitor if there is a history of peptic ulcer or aspirin-related dyspepsia), 40 mg of simvastatin, and blood pressure reduction. Evidence suggests that the lower the blood pressure, the lower the vascular risk, but this is a population at high risk of falls, and a lower as well as a higher blood pressure target seems sensible. We suggest 120/70–140/80 mmHg.

Dietary measures

- Fish contains omega-3 oils that may help to prevent heart disease, although this is not certain. Omega-3 oils may also be beneficial to the brain. Consumption of fish in the UK has fallen by 59% in the past 60 years. Population studies in the USA showed lower rates of dementia in people who ate oily fish at least once each week compared to those who rarely or never ate fish. Another study reported reduction in age related cognitive decline amongst those who ate fish twice weekly or more.
- Fruit and vegetables contain vitamins C and E; these are antioxidants, which may protect the brain from the deleterious effects of free radicals. Research on the effect of increased intake of these vitamins has produced mixed results; one study reported that high levels of vitamin C and E from fruit and vegetables was beneficial, but taking vitamin supplements was not. Large doses of vitamin E may increase mortality and interact with other medications.
- A healthy diet with plenty of fresh fruit and vegetables and oily fish twice a week may reduce the risk of dementia and is unlikely to be harmful. Vitamins and fish oil supplements are of no proven benefit and might be damaging.

Table 17.2 Summary of interventions to prevent stroke

Risk factor	Intervention	Evidence	Approximate relative risk of treatment
LIFESTYLE FACTORS			
Smoking	Stopping	Cohort studies	0.5 after 2 years
Inactivity	Moderate exercise	Cohort studies	0.5–0.7 in various studies
Salt intake	Reduction	Systematic review of RCTs, blood pressure end point	0.75 per 50 mmol Na/day
Obesity	Weight loss	Cohort studies	0.5 per 6 kg/m²
DRUG INTERVENTIONS			
Blood pressure	Drugs	Systematic reviews of RCTs	0.6 per 5–6 mmHg diastolic fall
Isolated systolic hypertension	Drugs	RCT	0.6 for 12 mmHg systolic fall
Cholesterol	Statin drugs	Systematic reviews of RCTs	0.75 (any vascular event)
Atrial fibrillation	Warfarin (INR 2–3)	Systematic reviews of RCTs	0.3
Atrial fibrillation	Aspirin	Systematic reviews of RCTs	0.8
TIA/minor stroke	Aspirin	Systematic reviews of RCTs	0.75
Post myocardial infarction	Warfarin	Systematic reviews of RCTs	0.5
SURGICAL INTERVENTIONS			
Symptomatic carotid stenosis (70–99%)	Surgery (vs medical)	RCT	0.5 (after 5 years inc. surgical mortality/ morbidity)*
Asymptomatic carotid stenosis (60–99%)	Surgery (vs medical)	RCT	0.5 (after 5 years inc. surgical mortality/ morbidity)*

RCT—randomized controlled trial.

* The effect of these interventions cannot be described by a single relative risk. Surgical morbidity produces an immediate hazard after which strokes accumulate more slowly in surgical patients. From Harwood, R. H., Huwez, F. and Good, D. 2005; *Stroke Care: a practical manual*. Oxford: OUP.

Box 17.1 Heart protection study and PROSPER trial—cholesterol reduction and antioxidant vitamin supplementation

- Participants were 20 536 people aged 40–80 years at high risk of vascular death by virtue of a prior vascular event (heart attack, stroke, or peripheral vascular disease), diabetes, or treated hypertension in men over 65 years old, and with a total cholesterol greater than 3.5 mmol/l.
- They were randomized to simvastatin 40 mg a day or placebo, and separately to a cocktail of antioxidant vitamins (E, C, and beta-carotene) in a 2 × 2 factorial design. Follow-up lasted 5 years.
- On average 85% of the intervention group took their statin, and 17% of the control group were given an out-of-trial statin. Total cholesterol was reduced on average by 1.2 mmol/l (LDL cholesterol by 1.0 mmol/l), but the difference between intervention and control dropped from 1.7 mmol/l in the first year to 0.8 mmol/l in the fifth year.
- 83% of participants continued their vitamin treatment. Plasma concentrations of vitamin E increased two-fold, vitamin C increased 30%, and beta-carotene increased four-fold.
- Relative risks on statin treatment were:
  - 0.87 (95% CI 0.81–0.94) for all-cause mortality (12.9% vs 14.7%)
  - 0.76 (0.72–0.81) for any major vascular event (19.8% vs 25.2%)
  - 0.75 (0.66–0.85) for any stroke (and TIA) (4.3% vs 5.7%).
- Relative risks on antioxidant vitamin treatment were:
  - 1.04 (95% CI 0.97–1.12) for all-cause mortality (14.1% vs 13.5%)
  - 1.00 (0.94–1.06) for any major vascular event (22.5% vs 22.5%)
  - 0.99 (0.87–1.12) for any stroke (and TIA) (5.0% vs 5.0%).
- Cognition was measured using a telephone interview, the modified Telephone Interview for Cognitive Status, TICS-m. Cognitive impairment was defined as a score lower than 22/39. Validity was confirmed as scores were worse with older age and with a history of stroke.
- In the statin trial, cognitive impairment at final follow-up was 23.7% vs 24.2%. Mean TICS-m score was 24.08 vs 24.06. 31 vs 31 developed diagnosed dementia, and 67 vs 60 some other psychiatric disorder. There was no interaction with age or history of stroke.
- In the vitamin trial, cognitive impairment at final follow-up was 23.4% vs 24.4%. Mean TICS-m score was 24.11 vs 24.04. 31 vs 31 developed diagnosed dementia and 62 vs 65 some other psychiatric disorder.
- Vascular mortality and morbidity was rapidly reduced by statin treatment, but not by antioxidant vitamins. Neither treatment had any effect on cognitive function over 5 years.
- The PROSPER trial of pravastatin amongst 5804 participants aged over 70, over 4 years follow-up, reported no difference in the MMSE or other specific cognitive function tests.

Lancet 2002; **360**: 7–22; 23–33; 1623–30

Box 17.2 The Syst-Eur blood pressure study

- Participants were 2418 men and women over 60 years of age with isolated systolic hypertension of 160–219 mmHg, but no cognitive impairment, randomized between active blood pressure lowering treatment or placebo.
- Active treatment was the calcium-channel blocker nitrendipine with enalapril and/or hydrochlorothiazide. Target blood pressure reduction was 20 mmHg or a systolic pressure of 150 mmHg. Active treatment produced a mean 8.3/3.8 mmHg reduction in BP compared with placebo.
- Median follow-up was 2 years. Cognitive function was assessed using the MMSE. Attempts were made to diagnose the pathological type of incident dementia.
- Relative risk of dementia on active treatment was 0.50 (95% CI 0.24–1.00) (3.8 vs 7.7/1000 patient-years). Mean MMSE score was not different between groups, however. Most cases were clinically diagnosed as Alzheimer's disease.
- This study was small in terms of the number of incident dementia cases (21 vs 11), it achieved only a small reduction in blood pressure, and the follow-up time was very short. Results could have arisen due to baseline imbalance or chance, or they may indicate a beneficial effect of reducing blood pressure.

Lancet 1998; **352**: 1347–51

Box 17.3 Women's Health Study Aspirin trial

- Participants were 6377 women aged over 65 years, with no evidence of baseline vascular disease or cognitive impairment, randomized to aspirin 100 mg on alternative days or placebo, and followed for a mean of 9.6 years (range 8–11 years).
- Cognitive function was tested using a battery of tests every 2 years after 5.6 years, administered by telephone. This included a telephone adaptation of the MMSE, a memory test, and a verbal fluency test.
- There were no differences in cognitive test results between the aspirin and placebo groups at any time point, apart from better verbal fluency (thought to be the most sensitive indicator of incipient cognitive decline) in the aspirin group at the final assessment only (relative risk of substantial decline 0.80, 95% CI 0.67–0.97).
- This was a negative study, but in a healthy cohort, and event rates may have been too small to show any effect. We cannot be sure of lack of effect in people with established vascular disease or multiple risk factors, or for intervention over a longer period of time. Notably, in subgroup analyses in this study, aspirin appeared to be more protective amongst smokers and those with high cholesterol.

BMJ 2007; **334**: 987–95

Box 17.4 Rotterdam study of alcohol and risk of dementia

- This was a cohort study of 7983 people aged over 55 years, who did not have dementia at baseline. Follow-up was for a mean of 6.0 years.
- Data on alcohol consumption was collected at baseline, by interview, as part of a food frequency questionnaire. Frequency, amount, and type of drink were recorded.
- Compared with no alcohol intake, consumption of 1–3 drinks per day was associated with a lower risk of incident dementia, regardless of type of alcoholic drink taken, and after adjustment for other risk factors:
  - relative risk was 0.58 (95% CI 0.38–0.90) for any dementia (197 cases, incidence rate 6.1/1000 person-years)
  - relative risk was 0.29 (95% CI 0.09–0.93) for vascular dementia (29 cases).
- Cohort studies are prone to information bias and residual confounding effects, so results are not conclusive. However, the effects of alcohol consumption are unlikely ever to be tested by randomized trial. Similar results have been reported from several other cohort studies.

Lancet 2002; **359**: 281–86

Box 17.5 Smoking and risk of dementia

- The British doctors study of 34 439 male doctors ascertained smoking status at baseline, and followed them up over 47 years, when 24 133 had died. Exposure status was periodically re-ascertained every 6–12 years.
- A dementia diagnosis was ascertained from death certificates (recorded in 473 cases). It is likely that dementia diagnoses were under-recorded by this method, but this will only have biased results if under-recording was different for smokers and non-smokers.
- Relative risk of dementia with smoking was:
  - 0.96 (95% CI 0.78–1.18) for all dementia
  - 0.99 (95% CI 0.78–1.25) for Alzheimer's disease.
- The Rotterdam Cohort of 6870 people over 55 years, without dementia at baseline, followed up for a mean 2.1 years (range 1.5–3.4) had better ascertainment of incident dementia. Participants were screened with the MMSE, then assessed by a neurologist. 146 new cases were detected.
- Relative risk of dementia with smoking, compared with never smoked, was:
  - 2.2 (95% CI 1.3–3.6) for all dementia
  - 2.3 (95% CI 1.3–4.1) for Alzheimer's disease.
- Risk was even greater (relative risk 4.6) in people without apolipoprotein ε4 allele, and for heavier smokers (relative risk 3.0 for current smokers with >20 pack years history).
- Previous reports of a protective effect of cigarette smoking on risk of dementia are unfounded.

BMJ 2000; **320**: 1097–1102; *Lancet* 1998; **351**: 1840–3

Box 17.6 Hormone (oestrogen) replacement therapy and dementia

- Participants were 4532 women aged over 65, initially free of dementia, randomized to oestrogen plus progestin or placebo. Mean follow-up was 4.1 years.
- Cognitive function was screened by annual modified MMSE tests. Possible cases of cognitive impairment had a full neuropsychological battery and clinical assessment for diagnosis and classification.
- Relative risk for women on treatment was:
  - 2.05 (95% CI 1.2–3.5) for 'probable dementia' (40 vs 21 cases)
  - 1.07 (95% CI 0.7–1.6) for mild cognitive impairment (63 vs 59 cases).
- Most cases were clinically diagnosed as Alzheimer's disease (20 oestrogen vs 12 placebo). Vascular dementia was seen in 5 vs 1 cases. 75 patients had strokes (39 vs 30), one of whom developed dementia.
- The trial was brief, and enrolled a healthy population in which the incidence of dementia was low. However, observational epidemiological suggestions that oestrogens were protective against dementia were unfounded.

JAMA 2003; **289**: 2651–62

Box 17.7 Folate supplementation and cognitive performance

- Participants were 818 men and women aged 50–70 with no initial dementia, raised plasma homocysteine (13–26 micromol/l), and normal vitamin B12, randomized to low dose (800 mcg daily) of folic acid or placebo. Follow-up was 3 years.
- Memory, attention, concept shifting, information processing, and verbal fluency were measured.
- Serum folate was raised seven-fold, plasma homocysteine decreased 26%.
- Rate of decline in memory, information processing speed, and concept shifting speed was lower in the folate group compared with the placebo group. A global cognitive score was better, but MMSE scores were the same between groups. The effect was equivalent to 1.5–4.7 years of age-related decline in performance.
- This study is far from establishing dementia prevention, but demonstrates convincing changes in specific cognitive functions, over a short period of time, in a highly selected population. It suggests that age-related decline in function is not immutable.

Lancet 2007; **369**: 208–16

Prevention of delirium and comorbidities

Chapter 3 p. 70 and Chapter 8 p. 207 give details of how to prevent delirium.

People with dementia are often frail and risk rapid deterioration in the face of intercurrent illness or injury. Subject to adequate and safe medicines management (compliance in particular), they are therefore good candidates for a range of prevention activity (📖 Table 17.3).

Table 17.3 Preventing comorbidity

Intervention	Subgroup	Comments
Influenza vaccination	All	
Influenza vaccination for (professional) carers	All	May be more effective than vaccinating patients
Pneumococcal vaccination	Chronic chest disease	
Calcium and vitamin D	Care home residents, osteoporosis, fracture history	No definite benefit for community-dwelling well elderly
Falls programme	History of falls, mild dementia	Reduces overt risks, but generally ineffective in moderate or severe dementia
Bisphosphonate (osteoporosis)	Fracture history	
Foot care	Diabetes	Reduces ulceration and amputation

Unnecessary disability, distress, and dependency

Some responses to problems make matters worse. Examples include over-prescription of sedative drugs, other forms of restraint, and immobility or reduced mobility.

Out-of-home respite, hospital stays, and holidays are also occasions of risk of distress or deterioration and require careful consideration and management.

'Adaptive' rehabilitation attempts to support people with dementia in the continued performance of activities of daily living, accepting that full independence will never be achieved, but preserving involvement and retention of some ability (📖 Chapter 8 p. 196).

Behavioural disturbance

Behavioural disturbance may be unavoidable, because without memory the world is a scary place and people fight back to defend themselves against perceived threats (📖 Chapter 4).

Analysis of disturbed behaviour often identifies misinterpretation or confrontation as an antecedent. With absent or defective reasoning ability, confrontation leads to escalation, anger, or aggression. 'Diversion not confrontation' helps avoid this.

Avoidance of new or unfamiliar environments, or careful preparation or support in them (such as a relative being given open visiting access in hospital), and maintenance of routines, helps.

Loss of 'personhood'

People with dementia are often not treated like people. They are ignored, talked over, not trusted, and may have every role, activity, or occupation systematically denied them by well meaning but overprotective carers.

Current best practice emphasizes maintaining the identity and role ('personhood') of the person with dementia. This means:
- Concentrating on the relationship between the person with dementia, the carer, and the support services.
- Fostering self-esteem and improving social confidence and communication.
- Allowing greater capacity to demonstrate agency and independence, including greater tolerance of apparent eccentricity or risk taking.

This requires coaching of family carers, and special training for professional staff. Conventional service provision usually entails the care delivered being dependent on the menu of tasks that the service provides, and is generally risk-averse. This model often fails to meet the subjective needs of either patient or carers. It undermines personhood by depersonalizing care. The person with dementia becomes a passive recipient. Caregivers and service providers are unable to form productive relationships with dementia sufferers due to lack of knowledge and skill on the part of the caregiver, shortage of time, and inconsistency in staff attending. People with dementia are often devalued or dehumanized by being ignored. Caregivers may detach themselves emotionally as a psychological coping strategy.

Appropriately trained care workers (e.g. home care or nurses) can avoid these pitfalls by building relationships over time, taking account of individual histories and preferences, and supporting involvement in everyday tasks.

Carer strain and morbidity

Being the main carer for someone with dementia is necessarily stressful. Some interventions aim to give support:

- Respite care: respite in the home ('sitting') is probably more acceptable and less disruptive than out of home respite, either in the form of adult day care or periods spent in care homes. However, different solutions work for different people, and some value periods of out of home respite.
- Community Mental Health Team involvement.
- Specialist Social Services intensive home support.
- Voluntary organizations (Alzheimer's Society, Carers Association).
- Times in hospital for other reasons.

Screening

Should we screen for cognitive impairment? In some settings (acute geriatric medical admissions, hip fracture and stroke patients, nursing and residential home residents) the prevalence of delirium and dementia will be such that a very low threshold for cognitive testing should be adopted, and this may approach 'screening'.

In general, there are good reasons for wanting to know about cognitive impairment if it is there, and a case can be made for older people being screened for cognitive problems (i.e. routinely and periodically tested in the absence of suggestive symptoms).

• Cognitive impairment is sometimes not noticed until there is a crisis.
• Cognitive impairment requires a diagnosis, especially if delirium is detected.
• A comprehensive assessment for other problems can be undertaken.
• Intervention may be possible to treat or mitigate problems, such as cholinesterase inhibitor drugs or treating comorbid depression.
• Plans can be made, especially wills and financial arrangements (such as Lasting Power of Attorney).
• In the expectation of future deterioration, regular (if not necessarily frequent) review or surveillance can be instituted.
• Problems can be anticipated (such as holidays or the possibility of decompensation during a hospital admission). With good planning, some, but not all, crises can be averted.
• Relatives and carers can be referred to, or made aware of, supporting services, either now or for the future.

There is a downside, which must be taken into account:
• Medical 'labelling' of problems can carry stigmatization and unneces-sary illness behaviour, such as disengagement or infantilization.
• Testing procedures may be seen as unnecessary or demeaning.
• Detecting minor problems, or false positive results, may cause anxiety or depression.
• False negative results can delay diagnosis or give false reassurance.

Several screening tools are available. The MMSE is best in complex older people. The AMT is suitable for widespread use in general medical or sur-gical settings. There are several possibilities for use in primary care apart from these, including the 6-CIT.

Remember that these are not diagnostic tools. A full score more or less excludes major problems, but people with pre-morbid high intelligence ('high baseline'), or fronto-temporal dementia, can score well despite significant problems. There is a wide differential diagnosis for low scores (📖 Chapter 2), including deafness, language problems, aphasia, and low educational attainment. They should be followed up by a fuller assessment, especially a cognitive history, and clinical mental state examination.

Comorbid conditions might also be valuably screened for. Vision, hearing, dental, and foot problems are all particularly common in frail older people, and people with dementia are not well catered for by standard services.

Genetic counselling

Apart from rare familial dementias, Huntington's chorea, and the risk of Down's syndrome in older mothers, genetic counselling plays little part in dementia prevention.

The vast majority of sufferers can be assured that heredity plays a minor role, and that they are unlikely to pass on a predisposition to future generations.

Genetic counselling is a major issue in Huntington's disease. It is an autosomal dominant condition, typically presenting in middle age. Offspring of an affected parent therefore have a 50% chance of developing the disease. Families will often know of the predisposition, but sporadic cases will usually present after the birth of children. If affected families choose to have children, assisted conception with donor gametes may be an option.

Decision-making and prevention

Benefits, burdens, autonomy/best interests, and justice should be considered as with any other intervention (🕮 Chapter 12).

Benefits should be clear but not overstated. Aspirin and statins in vascular disease prevention, for example, have a clear but small effect in reducing risk. Someone dying of cancer, or with limited life expectancy because of advanced neurodegenerative disease, is unlikely to benefit from multiple vascular prevention drugs. Conversely the 'benefit' of avoiding sedative medication is not realized if the drug genuinely reduced agitation or aggression, thereby enabling them to continue living at home.

Burdens include having to take tablets and any side effects. Polypharmacy is a real issue and has to be justified by anticipated benefits. As a general rule, any side effect is unacceptable in a preventative drug (health and well-being are compromised now to prevent something in the future that may never happen). If someone with dementia is not keen to take tablets, it will rarely be justified to make a fight of it for prevention purposes.

- If a person with dementia has capacity (🕮 Chapter 11), then they can decide whether to take any particular drug or not (or undergo any other intervention). Serving someone's best interests does not mean medical paternalism. Even if they lack capacity, involving them in deciding and taking account of current wishes remain important, if not overriding, factors to take into account. Similarly, relatives' and carers' views should be considered.

- Justice means not discriminating against someone because of age or disability, and using resources efficiently. Someone should not be deprived of preventative intervention just because of dementia, but this is not the only factor and limited life expectancy, side effects, or disinclination to take tablets are perfectly good reasons for withdrawing preventative drugs.

Summary

1. Most prevention is based on risk factor epidemiology, confirmed by randomized controlled trials. The epidemiology is relatively underdeveloped, but to date there is no confirmed intervention to prevent AD, DLB, or FTD. Heavy alcohol intake is harmful, and smoking is not protective.
2. Vascular disease is in part preventable, but the evidence that vascular prevention can reduce cognitive impairment is weak.
3. A broader view of prevention considers adverse consequences, complications, and comorbidities, as well as disease prevention. Good management contributes to a reduction in these (although the distinction between prevention and care is blurred).
4. Amongst elderly general medical inpatients, delirium can be reduced by best practice nursing and medicine.
5. In some settings, screening for dementia is justified.

Chapter 18

Outcome in dementia

Outcome in dementia

There are currently nearly 700 000 people in the UK with dementia.

This figure is forecast to increase to nearly 1 million by 2021 (38% rise) and 1.75 million by 2051 (150% rise).

Rates of increase of dementia are even higher in the developing world. Numbers in developed countries are forecast to increase by 100% between 2001 and 2040, but by more than 300% in India, China, south Asia, and the western Pacific region.

Epidemiology

Prevalence *is the proportion of people in any population who have a particular disorder.*

E.g. 'The prevalence of dementia in people aged 85–89 in the UK is 22%.'

Incidence *is the number of new cases arising each year in a population.*

E.g. 'The incidence of dementia in developed countries in people aged 85–89 is 5.3%.'

Numbers of people with dementia may increase due to three causes:
• Dementia becoming more common (i.e. an increase in the incidence of dementia).
• People with dementia living longer (an increase in survival).
• An ageing population (more people of an age to be at risk of dementia).

Dementia at a given age is not becoming more common. Long-term studies in Scandinavia and North America have shown little change in age-specific dementia rates. Survival in dementia is rising as a result of improvements in care. The total number of cases of dementia is increasing mainly due to the ageing of the population. The rates of dementia at different ages from a recent English survey are shown in Fig. 18.1 and Fig. 18.2.

There are no data on the prevalence of dementia in ethnic minority groups in the UK. There are relatively few older people from Asia, Africa, and the Caribbean in this country now. Dementia will become more common in these groups as the population ages. In the USA, Hispanic and African-American men have higher prevalence of dementia, probably because hypertension and diabetes, which are risk factors for dementia, are more common in these ethnic groups. Studies in the Far East show a change in the predominant type of dementia being diagnosed. In the 1980s most cases of dementia were attributed to vascular disease, whereas in the 1990s Alzheimer's disease was more commonly reported. It is not clear whether this reflects a change in diagnostic practice after the emergence of specific therapy for Alzheimer's disease or improved treatment of vascular risk factors.

About one-third of people with dementia in the UK are currently thought to be living in care homes. The only national survey undertaken (in Canada in 1994) found that half of people with dementia were in institutional care. Clearly these rates will depend on the threshold for detecting dementia.

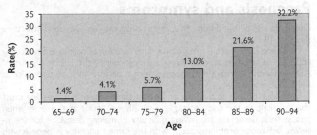

Fig. 18.1 Prevalence of dementia with advancing age.

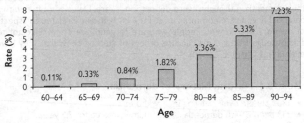

Fig. 18.2 Incidence of dementia.

Prognosis and symptoms

Dementia is a condition that gets progressively worse with time (📖 Box 18.1).

In AD and DLB there is progressive deterioration of cognitive functioning and skills in activities of daily living, although during the first few years of AD, even without treatment, improvement in performance on tests such as the MMSE may occur.

Behaviour problems may occur early in the disorder, but they are most characteristic in the middle stages, typically appearing at the time when people with dementia are having difficulty in making decisions for themselves. Behaviour problems occur with the same frequency in people with AD, VaD, or mixed Alzheimer's and vascular dementia, but are more frequent in DLB.

About 25% of people with AD develop depression during the course of their dementia, although severe depression is rare. Delusions, often with a paranoid flavour, are common; most frequently they are related to aspects of memory impairment. People who are forgetful are often reluctant to acknowledge this and may accuse others of stealing items that they have mislaid (📖 Chapter 2 p. 30).

Box 18.1 Natural history of dementia

- 1800 people over 75 living in Stockholm.
- 233 people with dementia at outset, followed up for 7.5 years.
- Progression:
  - 50 months—two-thirds had moderate dementia
  - 80 months—80% had moderate dementia.
- Mortality:
  - 3 years—40% dead
  - 5 years—70% dead.
- Admission to care:
  - 40 months—50% in institutional care
  - 60 months—80% in institutional care.

Aguero-Torres, H. et al. *JAGS 1998*; **46**: 444–52

Natural history of BPSD

Three distinctive patterns have been described:

A. Single episode, remitting before death.
• Typical symptoms:
  • increase in eating
  • increase in walking
  • needing to be brought home.

B. Single episode, persisting until death.
• Typical symptoms:
  • diminished eating
  • verbal aggression
  • aggressive resistance
  • physical aggression.

C. Several episodes with periods of remission.
(No particular associated symptoms.)

Survival

Dementia shortens the lifespan.

The best predictor of early death in dementia is comorbid poor physical health, specifically:
- Diabetes.
- Heart failure.
- Ischaemic heart disease.
- Gait disturbance.

Other indicators of poor prognosis:
- More severe disease at time of presentation.
- Rapid progression in first year after diagnosis.
- Male sex.
- Wandering.

Early behaviour disturbance (apart from wandering) does not shorten life expectancy. There are no differences in outcome by social class.

Recent research in community based cohorts suggests that the average time from diagnosis to death is:
- 3–4 years for men.
- 3.5–6 years for women.

Differences between the sexes diminish with increasing age. Diagnosis at a younger age is associated with longer survival:
- 10.7 years for onset 65–69.
- 5.4 years onset 70–79.
- 4.3 years onset 80–89.

People with vascular dementia have shorter life expectancy than those with Alzheimer's disease, probably as a result of their systemic cardiovascular disease.

Summary

1. Dementia is becoming more common (increased prevalence) because of better survival and the ageing of the population
2. Symptoms get progressively worse with time. The rate of progression varies widely between people. On average after 5–7 years 80% progress to at least moderate symptoms and 80% will be admitted to care homes.
3. Behavioural problems typically appear in mid-disease and change over time. Perhaps half remit; highlighting the need for regular monitoring and reassessment.
4. Average survival 3–4 years for men, and 3.5–6 years for women, but varies with age at diagnosis (11 years for onset 65–69, 5 years onset 70–79, 4 years onset 80–89)

Index